CARDIAC REMODELING

MOLECULAR MECHANISMS, TREATMENT AND CLINICAL IMPLICATIONS

CARDIOLOGY RESEARCH AND CLINICAL DEVELOPMENTS

CARDIOLOGY RESEARCH AND CLINICAL DEVELOPMENTS

CARDIAC REMODELING

MOLECULAR MECHANISMS, TREATMENT AND CLINICAL IMPLICATIONS

JERALD SHERMAN

EDITOR

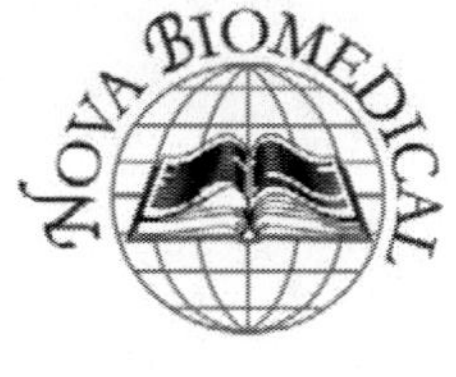

New York

NOTICE TO THE READER

Library of Congress Cataloging-in-Publication Data

Library of Congress Control Number: 2015956840

ISBN: 978-1-63484-270-9

Published by Nova Science Publishers, Inc. † New York

CONTENTS

PREFACE

Cardiovascular diseases are the leading cause of death in almost 40% of patients suffering from end stage renal disease (ESRD). Cardiomyopathy and ischemic heart disease are the most frequent causes of cardiac death. The risk of cardiovascular mortality in dialysis patients is 10 to 20 times greater than the general population, particularly in younger patients, taking into account that the relative risk decreases with age. Left ventricular hypertrophy (LVH) is the most common cardiac abnormality in chronic kidney disease (CKD), and the survival risk ratio in such patients is independent. This book examines the molecular mechanisms, treatments and clinical implication of cardiac remodeling. The first chapter discusses risk factors for cardiovascular disease in patients on continuous ambulatory peritoneal dialysis. The following chapters examine the impacts tropomyosin, vitamin D, and coffee have on cardiac remodeling.

Chapter 1 – Cardiovascular diseases are the leading cause of mortality in patients with end stage renal disease (ESRD). The aim of study was to evaluate changes on the left ventricular and carotid arteries (CCA) in patients with ESRD at baseline and 18 months after starting the peritoneal dialysis (PD) treatment in order to investigate the contribution of traditional risk factors to uremia-related factors and risk factors specific for peritoneal dialysis.

Fifty PD patients were included in a prospective longitudinal study, with laboratory, echocardiography, and CCA ultrasound parameters evaluation at the start of peritoneal dialysis and after the follow-up period of 18 months.

Left ventricular hypertrophy (LVH) was present baseline in 78%, and after 18 months in 60% PD patients. Atherosclerosis in the CCA was observed in 44% of baseline and after 18 months of PD treatment in 26% of patients. It was confirmed that low-density lipoproteins (LDL), troponin and C reactive protein (CRP) were independent risk factors for the development of LVH. Inverse relationship with LVH showed residual renal function, proteinuria, and nitric oxide (NO). The level of NO in serum was significantly increased during the 18 months of follow-up (p < 0.001), while the level of endothelin-1 (ET-1) in the same period fell significantly (p < 0.001). Independent predictors of intima media thickness CCA in PD patients were homocysteine, CRP, LDL, lipoprotein (a), product CaxP, ET-1 and proteinuria. Patients with LVH and atherosclerotic changes in the CCA had a lower dialysis adequacy, while the transport characteristics of the peritoneum in most patients were in the range of high-average and high transporters.

The presence of cardiovascular remodeling in ESRD highlights the importance of identifying and correcting changes in cardiovascular risk factors present in ESRD, as well as during the renal replacement therapy.

Chapter 2 – Tropomyosin (Tpm), an α-helical coiled coil protein, is an integral component of the thin filament in the cardiac muscle sarcomere. Striated muscle contraction is regulated through a calcium (Ca^{2+}) –dependent mechanism involving Tpm, troponin, actin, and myosin. Tpm occupies a unique structural position by serving as the intermediary effector that repositions itself when Ca^{2+} binds troponin. When Ca^{2+} binds to troponin C, a conformational change occurs allowing Tpm to shift its position and move away from the myosin binding sites on the sarcomeric actin filament, resulting in the myosin head binding to actin and leading to muscle contraction. There are three primary striated muscle Tpm isoforms generated from distinct genes. Their laboratory has focused on understanding the function of these Tpm isoforms. Studies from their laboratory demonstrate that increased expression of the embryonic cardiac β-Tpm isoform can lead to a dramatic hypertrophic cardiomyopathic condition. In addition, mutations in Tpm are associated with human hypertrophic (HCM) and dilated (DCM) cardiomyopathies. In order to investigate HCM and DCM conditions caused by Tpm mutations, the authors generated animal models that incorporate these HCM and DCM mutations. An advantage in using transgenic mice is that the endogenous α-Tpm isoform decreases its expression in proportion with increased expression of exogenous Tpm expression through both post-transcriptional and translational regulatory mechanisms. The authors find incorporation of these HCM- and DCM-causing Tpm mutations in transgenic mice lead to cardiac remodeling that resembles the pathological changes found in hypertrophic or dilated cardiomyopathy patients; in addition, physiological alterations also occur in the diseased murine myocardium that reflect the functional abnormalities found in HCM and DCM patients. Furthermore, they found that modulation of the phosphorylation status of Tpm can also trigger cardiac remodeling . Interestingly, their studies show the aberrant phenotypes that are generated by Tpm mutations can also be "rescued" through modifications in Tpm which affect the myofilament's response to Ca^{2+}. These studies demonstrate that Tpm plays a unique role in its ability to not only cause morphological and functional alterations in the diseased heart, but it can also reverse the pathological and physiological remodeling that occurs during cardiomyopathic conditions.

Chapter 3 – The micronutrient vitamin D has long been appreciated for its role in the homeostasis of bone and in the prevention of rickets. Many studies have shown that vitamin D supplementation may also be effective in the prevention and treatment of disorders of the immune system and inflammation, as well as treatment of diseases such as diabetes, cancer and osteoarthritis. There is growing evidence sustaining an important role for vitamin D on heart health as well.

Recent studies have demonstrated that vitamin D deficiency is very common in patients affected by chronic renal disease or heart failure, and it is associated with poor outcome among these patients. Heart failure has its origins rooted in adverse structural, biochemical and molecular remodeling of myocardium. Vitamin D receptors (VDR) are widespread in the myocardial cellular constituents, including cardiomyocytes, thus justifying an in-depth analysis of how vitamin D accounts for the causes and consequences of adverse heart remodeling. Vitamin D effects are translated at the cellular level through the activation of the specific nuclear receptor by the active metabolite of vitamin D, 1,25-dihydroxyvitamin D. Vitamin D is a negative regulator of the renin-angiotensin system and acts to reduce hypertrophic, apoptotic and pro-fibrotic gene expression. Mechanistic insights were gained mainly by experimental studies on VDR-deficient mice, which develop hypertension and adverse cardiac remodeling mediated via the renin-angiotensin system. In addition, studies on mouse models of cardiomyocyte-specific deletion of VDR demonstrated an increase in myocyte size and left ventricular hypertrophy in the conditional knockout.

Given the clinical impact of adverse ventricular remodeling, this review summarizes current knowledge on vitamin D and its biology in heart failure to extend their understanding of factors that may act against ventricular hypertrophy and abnormal geometry.

Chapter 4 – It is well known that moderate coffee intake inhibits the development of cardiovascular diseases in clinical settings. However, the effect of chlorogenic acid (CGA), one of the major polyphenol constituents of coffee beans, on the disease is yet to be elucidated. This article reviews the effect of CGA on myocardial remodeling. Firstly, the authors reviewed the effects of CGA on human cardiovascular diseases. Several studies indicated that CGA might decrease the clinical risk of cardiovascular diseases via anti-hypertensive and anti-endothelial dysfunction. Next, the authors demonstrated that CGA could improve pathological remodeling through the suppression of myocardial cell infiltration and fibrosis in animal models. Their findings and previous data suggest that the CGA treatment may have beneficial effects on the progression of myocardial remodeling.

In: Cardiac Remodeling
Editor: Jerald Sherman

ISBN: 978-1-63484-270-9
© 2016 Nova Science Publishers, Inc.

Chapter 1

RISK FACTORS FOR CARDIOVASCULAR DISEASE IN PATIENTS ON CONTINUOUS AMBULATORY PERITONEAL DIALYSIS

Damir Rebić[1,*] *and Velma Rebić*[2]
[1]Clinic for Nephrology, University Clinical Center of Sarajevo,
Bosnia and Herzegovina
[2]Medical Faculty University of Sarajevo, Bosnia and Herzegovina

ABSTRACT

Cardiovascular diseases are the leading cause of mortality in patients with end stage renal disease (ESRD). The aim of study was to evaluate changes on the left ventricular and carotid arteries (CCA) in patients with ESRD at baseline and 18 months after starting the peritoneal dialysis (PD) treatment in order to investigate the contribution of traditional risk factors to uremia-related factors and risk factors specific for peritoneal dialysis.

Fifty PD patients were included in a prospective longitudinal study, with laboratory, echocardiography, and CCA ultrasound parameters evaluation at the start of peritoneal dialysis and after the follow-up period of 18 months.

---

[*] Corresponding author: Damir Rebić, M.D., Ph.D. Clinic for nephrology, UCC Sarajevo 71000 Sarajevo, Bosnia and Herzegovina, tel.: + 387 33 297043, fax: + 387 33 297925, e-mail: damir.rebic@gmail.com.

Left ventricular hypertrophy (LVH) was present baseline in 78%, and after 18 months in 60% PD patients. Atherosclerosis in the CCA was observed in 44% of baseline and after 18 months of PD treatment in 26% of patients. It was confirmed that low-density lipoproteins (LDL), troponin and C reactive protein (CRP) were independent risk factors for the development of LVH. Inverse relationship with LVH showed residual renal function, proteinuria, and nitric oxide (NO). The level of NO in serum was significantly increased during the 18 months of follow-up ($p < 0.001$), while the level of endothelin-1 (ET-1) in the same period fell significantly ($p < 0.001$). Independent predictors of intima media thickness CCA in PD patients were homocysteine, CRP, LDL, lipoprotein (a), product CaxP, ET-1 and proteinuria. Patients with LVH and atherosclerotic changes in the CCA had a lower dialysis adequacy, while the transport characteristics of the peritoneum in most patients were in the range of high-average and high transporters.

The presence of cardiovascular remodeling in ESRD highlights the importance of identifying and correcting changes in cardiovascular risk factors present in ESRD, as well as during the renal replacement therapy.

1. INTRODUCTION

Cardiovascular diseases are the leading cause of death in almost 40% of patients suffering from end stage renal disease (ESRD). Cardiomyopathy and ischemic heart disease are the most frequent causes of cardiac death [1]. The risk of cardiovascular mortality in dialysis patients is 10 to 20 times greater than the general population, particularly in younger patients, taking into account that the relative risk decreases with age. Left ventricular hypertrophy (LVH) is the most common cardiac abnormality in chronic kidney disease (CKD), and the survival risk ratio in such patients is independent [2].

Epidemiological and clinical studies have shown that damage of the large arteries presents the main risk factor, which adds to the high mortality rate in patients suffering from ESRD. Macrovascular disease develops quickly in uremic patients, and it is responsible for high incidence of ischemic heart disease [3]. Although most such changes can be the consequence of atherosclerotic obstructive lesions, in 25-30% of patients, the origin of the blood vessel damage is non-atherosclerotic, and is mostly tied to micro vascular disease or fibroelastic thickening of the aorta, which further reduces arterial compliance and causes non-atherosclerotic remodeling. Both cardiac and vascular disorders share several common, connected pathophysiological mechanisms [4].

Cardiac Disease and ESRD

The leading causes of death in patients with ESRD are cardiac complications, with over 50% mortality of uremic patients on dialysis. Cardiac mortality is reflected in high incidence of congestive heart insufficiency, cardiomyopathy, pericarditis, hypertension, sudden death and, in most cases, ischemia and myocardial infarction. Cardiac disease is very common at the very start of dialysis treatment of CKD, and as such has a high incidence with chronic dialysis patients [4].

Cardiac disease in uremic patients most commonly develops because of cardiomyopathy, and/or, coronary heart disease. The term, uremic cardiomyopathy pertains to heterogenic (systolic and diastolic dysfunction) and multifactorial pathology, which appears during chronic renal failure (CRF), and can be registered by echocardiography as left ventricular hypertrophy, left ventricular dilatation and functional left ventricular disorder. These diseases are often present in dialysis patients [4].

Uremic Cardiomyopathy

In the general population, pathological LVH is connected to poor survival prognosis, the development of diastolic dysfunction, arrhythmias and cardiac failure progression. A similar state is present with predialysis, as well as dialysis patients. Although the terms used to describe this condition overlap, uremic cardiomyopathy marks the influence of reduced renal function on functional cardiac capability [5].

Epidemiological studies show that the primary manifestation of uremic cardiomyopathy is LVH. Reduced renal function in different stages of arrest, combined with cardiac diseases, most often causes the development of uremic cardiomyopathy. Go and assoc., in a study on a large number of examinees, determined that the reduction of glomerular filtration rate (GFR) by 50%, increases the overall risk of death by 5 times [6].

The treatment of ESRD by kidney transplantation severely reduces the risk of cardiovascular death, but with persistence of some mortality risks. Zoccali and assoc. work shows that short term dialysis patients have a better prognosis and survival concerning cardiovascular diseases post kidney transplantation. The same authors determined that LVH is an independent factor of cardiovascular risk, connected to significant survival rate reduction [7].

LVH pathogenesis in uremic cardiomyopathy remains uncertain. Taking into account the high frequency of hypertension in patients with difficult chronic renal disease, one of the hypotheses is that LVH occurs as a product of blood pressure encumbrance. In patients with diabetic nephropathy, blood pressure, as an independent risk factor, leads to the increase of left ventricular mass (LVM), as well as the LV mass index (LVMI).

The application of blood pressure drugs, as well as dialysis treatment successfully reduces ventricular mass [8], and so, this treatment is used in normotensive patients. The application of angiotensin converting enzyme (ACE) inhibitors reduces left ventricular mass in dialysis patients, previously normotensive. Larsen and assoc. have shown that left ventricular wall size is reduced in patients on intensive, continuous and daily dialysis, over the course of a year, unlike those patients who had intermittent dialysis three times a week, despite similar systolic blood pressure values [9].

Another potential cause of uremic cardiomyopathy is volume encumbrance, which can cause the development of eccentric LVH, by increasing left ventricular end diastolic diameter (LVEDD). The reduction of interdialytic mass correlates with LVMI reduction, but LVH can persist, irrelevant of LVMI normalization [10].

Another hypothesis on the etiology of uremic cardiomyopathy is that the accumulation of hypertrophic growth factor, connecter to ESRD, initiates signal activation independent of mechanical stress, which leads to cardiac pathology progression. Several matters can modulate cardiac growth and function, which are accumulated in ESRD patients, primarily endothelin-1, parathyroid hormone, tumor necrosis factor-α, leptin, interleukin-1α, and interleukin-6 [11].

Left Ventricular Hypertrophy

The prevalence of LVH is high among patients suffering from ESRD. Structural changes appear in the early stages of kidney function damage. In prospective research, just prior to the start of renal replacement therapy, 74% of patients had LVH, with a high LVMI, as an independent mortality predictor after two years of dialysis treatment. Up to 80% of dialysis patients have increased LVM [12]. The increase of LVM in ESRD patients can be caused by an increase of LVEDD as a result of volume encumbrance, the increase of left ventricular wall thickening, and the combination of characteristics of both eccentric and concentric LVH. The precise distinction of LVH between eccentric and concentric is sometimes difficult in hemodialysis patients, because of cyclical variations of extra cellular fluid and humeral balance. The internal dimensions of LV are under the influence of the volume status, and the decrease of blood volume during dialysis reduces LV diameter, causing "acute" changes in the relative thickness of the left ventricular wall. In stable patients with compensated hypertrophy, systolic function remains within normal boundaries, while diastolic charging often varies [13].

LVH is an adaptive response to increased heart rate. LVH is both damaging and beneficial at the same time. The benefits are tied to the number of sarcomeres and the increase of heart function capability, which allows for energy conservation. Such an effect sustains normal systolic function during the initial, compensated, or "adaptive" phase of LVH development. Continued stress gradually leads to an "inappropriate" hypertrophic response. In this phase of LVH, a loss of balance between energy consumption and production occurs in the activated myocardial cells, which eventually results in chronic energy deficiency and accelerated myocyte death [14].

The increase of extracellular matrix and collagen content makes the functional competence of heart contractions sustainable, however, at the expense of weakened diastolic charging. LVH usually occurs as a response to initiated mechanical stress. Pressure encumbrance results in parallel addition of new sarcomeres, with a disproportionate increase in LV wall thickness and a normal ventricular diameter (concentric hypertrophy). Volume encumbrance primarily results in the addition of new sarcomeres in series, and a secondary order of new sarcomeres parallel, which, again leads to the increase of LV diameter, with an increase of wall thickness (eccentric hypertrophy). The development and markings of LVH are under the influence of several factors such as age, gender, and race, a co-existing disease, such as diabetes, systemic disease, or kidney failure [3].

Vascular Remodeling and ESRD

The changes in the vascular system of uremic patients are attributed to a synergistic effect of numerous factors, such as dyslipidemia, prothrombotic factors, anemia, hypertension, increased oxidative stress, hyperparathyroidism, synthesis disorder homocysteine and nitric oxide, endothelial dysfunction, as well as LV remodeling, which leads to the modification of structural and functional cardiac and vascular characteristics.

Pathophysiology of the Changes in the Vascular System in ESRD Patients

Pathophysiological changes of the arterial system in ESRD, as well as in the general population, are heterogeneous etiologies. Atherosclerosis (plaque growth) and arterial remodeling are, first and foremost, connected to aging (arteriosclerosis) and hemodynamic changes. Atherosclerosis and arterial occlusive changes are the most common causes of cardiovascular morbidity in patients on renal replacement therapy. Occlusive changes mostly involve the median involvement of large intake arteries, and cardiac weakness. Peripheral artery disease and cerebrovascular incidents occupy an important place in the etiology of mortalities of dialysis patients. Meuss and associates' research has shown a high occurrence of atherosclerosis in CKD patients, and established a hypothesis of accelerated atherosclerosis in CKD [15].

However, the questions, whether atherogenesis in CRD patients is accelerated, and is the nature of the atherosclerotic plaque in CRD patients similar to the general population, remain unanswered. Ultrasound studies have shown a much greater occurrence of calcified plaques in ESRD patients, than in a control group of the general population of a similar age, where soft atherosclerotic plaques were found more often [16]. Renal failure alone leads to the creation of numerous atherogenic factors, which are specific to the uremic environment, such as dyslipidemia, calcium-phosphorus conditional changes, malnutrition in patients, and cytosine activation. These uremic factors are only an addition to previously observed and verified risk factors, such as age, hypertension, smoking, diabetes, male gender, and insulin resistance in subjects with preserved renal function. Many patients obtain significant vascular lesions at the very start of dialysis treatment, and in many patients, particularly older ones, generalized atherosclerosis can be the main cause of renal failure.

Hypertension is a common complication in ESRD, and the connection between high blood pressure and arterial lesions has been established in chronic renal patients. Current research shows that rigorous controls of hypertension in early CRD stages lead to severely reduced instances of myocardial ischemia, after the commencement of dialysis treatment [17]. Besides atherosclerosis and the presence of atherosclerotic plaques, the arterial system in ESRD patients undergoes a process of remodeling, which is presented by dilation, and artery intimal-medial thickness, which particularly affects medium, large, elastic capacitive arteries, such as the aorta and the common carotid arteries. Arterial remodeling is less common in smaller, peripheral arteries, such as the radial arteries. In ESRD patients, this remodeling is connected to arterial rigidity, primarily caused by the increase of the elastic incremental module (Einc), which coats the internal structure of the vascular wall with thick material properties. The effect of increased Einc is primarily in the attenuated increase of arterial diameter. As a consequence of this change, arterial diameter is commonly kept in the boundaries of normal values, but the extensibility of the capacitive artery is reduced. In uremic patients, abnormal arterial rigidity should primarily be observed in younger patients, because in the older population the effects of age on arterial rigidity dominate the effects of uremia [18]. Many elderly ESRD patients can manifest vascular nephropathy, but in this instance arterial changes primarily reflect primary arterial disease, and not uremic involvement.

Clinical Readings of Arterial Remodeling

Arterial changes in ESRD patients are responsible for increased systolic and pulse rate pressure. In the general population, pulse rate pressure has shown itself to be a strong risk predictor in the development of coronary disease, and vascular complications. By applying logistical regression and Cox analysis in dialysis patients, Blacher and associates determined that aortic extensibility, measured by the PWV aorta, is a strong and independent predictor of cardiovascular, but also combined mortality. PWV is a complex parameter of arterial stricter integration and internal elastic properties, measured using the Moens-Korteweg equation ($PWV^2 = Eh/2rp$, where E is an elasticity module (Einc), r is radius, h is wall thickness, and p is liquid density). Based on such measurements and data analysis, Blacher and associates have determined that the main "hemodynamic" risk factor in cardio vascular and other mortality causes in ESRD is the elasticity and arterial dilation module, which is, generally speaking, an arterial disease [19].

Dialysis treatment by itself does not improve arterial extensibility. In older hypertensive nonuremic patients, long term antihypertensive therapy and good blood pressure control leads to the regression of arterial ventricular hypertrophy and the improvement of the arterial system in general, particularly the elastic properties of the arteries. So far such controlled, long term studies have not been undertaken in ESRD patients. During the last few years, several controlled studies have been directed at the study of the effects of antihypertensive drugs on large artery function and morphology in ESRD patients, mostly on hemodialysis (HD), while there has still been no major research in peritoneal dialysis patients (PD). For HD patients it has been proven that calcium channel blockers reduce blood pressure, as well as the PSW aorta and femoral artery. ACE inhibitors have had the same effect of arterial extensibility. However these studies have not answered the question: has the improvement of the elastic properties of arteries occurred through well controlled blood pressure, or through the regression of structural arterial wall changes, in the sense of reduced remodeling and improved characteristics of the internal vascular wall [20].

Peritoneal Dialysis and Cardiovascular Diseases

Peritoneal dialysis (PD) is a dialysis treatment in which one to three liters of commercially made dialysis solution is inserted into the peritoneal cavity. Diffusion and osmosis takes place through the peritoneum, a semi-porous membrane, which aids the exchange of molecules and functions as a natural filter. Fluid is effused out of the abdominal space, by which toxic metabolism products and excess water are removed. The most practiced form of peritoneal dialysis is continuous ambulatory peritoneal dialysis (CAPD), where the abdominal cavity is constantly filled with dialysis solution, which is replaced every 4-6 hours, so that four to five daily replacements are conducted with 1 to 3 liters of dialysis solution.

Cardiovascular diseases are an almost unavoidable result in CAPD treated patients, and are the leading cause of death, with a 5 to 20 times greater occurrence than in the general population.

Cardiomyopathies in uremic CAPD patients occur as a consequence of pressure encumbrance, volume encumbrance or both. Increased blood pressure leads to concentric LVH, while volume encumbrance causes its dilation. Cardiomyopathies are seen through systolic and diastolic function disorders. Systolic weakness (reduced cardiac contractility) is a consequence of myocyte death during uremia, a significant contributor to ischemic, atherogenic and nonatherogenic cardiac diseases. Diastolic dysfunction reflects disorders in left ventricular charging, caused by late relaxation of the rigid, fibrous ventricular wall.

In CAPD patients, LVH, through the increase of sarcomere numbers, and the thickening of the ventricular wall, has the property of maintaining myocardial wall stability on extension stress and energy preservation. It also causes reduced capillary density in the grown cardiac mass, thus reducing coronary reserves and perfusion of the subendocardial myocardial level [21].

A series of other cardiac abnormalities are present in PD patients: interstitial myocardial fibrosis dependent on hyperthyroidism, reduced cardiac perfusion reserves through structural and functional changes of the heart muscle arteries and a reduced capillary density within the myocardium, a disturbed myocardial metabolism, which acts through synergy with a reduced blood flow, because of the maintaining of ischemic tolerance (a reduced response to β-adrenergic stimulation, inadequate control of intercellular concentrations of calcium ions, a disrupted glucose intake dependent on insulin, and an abnormal oxidation metabolism of the heart muscle) [22]. Clinical consequences of this produced cardiomyopathy are cardiac insufficiency, ischemic heart disease, arrhythmias, and mortality.

Atherosclerosis presents a significant cause of increased cardiovascular morbidity and mortality in PD patients. Even though atherosclerosis is not the only cause of this, it presents the main risk factor for cardiovascular complications in peritoneal dialysis treated patients. Structural carotid artery (CCA) changes, intima media thickness (IMT), can be considered a "mirror" of systemic atherosclerosis [23].

Risk factors of cardiovascular diseases in peritoneal dialysis patients can be divided into general factors, ESRD connected factors, and factors specific to peritoneal dialysis.

Traditional Risk Factors in Patients on Peritoneal Dialysis

Hypertension, smoking, hyperlipidemia, obesity, and diabetes are all risk factors which are connected to cardiovascular diseases in general populations, but also in PD patients, and are categorized into so-called traditional risk factors.

1. Arterial Hypertension

Arterial hypertension is very common in chronic kidney (CKD) disease patients and is connected to increased risk of cardiovascular death [24]. Hypertension is often present in peritoneal dialysis patients. According to the results of an Italian multicentric study, 88% of 504 patients treated with PD suffer from arterial hypertension, with antihypertensive therapy included. Arterial hypertension in PD patients is usually connected to volume encumbrance [25]. In a report by the UK renal registry in 2008, it is stated that in a larger number of patients treated with hemodialysis the targeted blood pressure was achieved, as opposed to PD patients (45% to 33%) [26].

However, unlike the general population of dialysis treated patients, the connection between high blood pressure and mortality is not so pronounced.

Hypertension strongly correlates with LVH, which is often found in CKD. Almost 70% of patients at the beginning of dialysis therapy suffer from an echocardiography recognizable LVH. According to research done by Coen and associates, LVH is more potent in long-term PD patients than in hemodialysis patients, most likely because of inadequate volume control [27].

2. Atherosclerosis

It has been proven that arterial rigidity, which is usually estimated by pulse wave velocity on the aorta, the quantity of CCA IMT, and also by peak systolic velocity in the systole on the CCA, is a useful predictor of cardiovascular morbidity and mortality in the general population, and as such, in patients suffering from CKD [28].

Zoccali and associates, through their research, have determined that in a large group of patients suffering from CKD, the rigidity of large arteries was independently connected with age, blood pressure, as well as other risk factors for the development of cardiovascular diseases. The presence of vascular calcifications has shown itself to be one of the most prominent factors connected to arterial rigidity. However, relevant studies in PD patients are relatively small and have numerous limitations [29].

3. Tobacco Smoking

Smoking is not only a risk factor for the development of cardiovascular diseases, but is also connected to the risk of developing CKD, defined as the reduction GFR at <45ml/min/1.73 m². In a large study from Norway, long term smoking of over 20 cigarettes a day is connected to a 1.52 times increased relative risk of CKD occurrence [30, 31]. However, it is relatively unknown whether smoking increases the risk of cardiovascular death in PD patients. A small study on diabetic PD patients found no effects of smoking on the risk of CV death, although a series of studies showed that smoking, or a history of smoking, is an independent risk factor on increased morbidity and mortality [31]. These apparent differences can be framed through the presence of other risk factors in some populations, which can supersede the effects of smoking in various multivariable analyses.

4. Obesity

Obesity is a risk factor for the development of CV diseases in the general population, but is also connected to an increased risk factor for the development of CKD [31].

The results of studies performed on PD patients have not been consistent about the influence of obesity on survival rates. The results of some studies showed that obesity is connected to better survival rates [32], while other studies have discovered that there is a connection between obesity and increased mortality risk. A prospective, time limited analysis in 688 PD patients showed that only those with a BMI <18.5 have an increased risk of CV death. High BMI had no protective effective, but was also not connected to reduced survival risk [33].

5. Dyslipidemia

Dyslipidemia is known as a traditional risk factor for cardiovascular diseases in the general population, as well as in dialysis patients. Several observational studies have shown that the values of cholesterol and low-density lipoprotein (LDL) are among the most significant independent cardiovascular morbidity and mortality factors [34]. Patients with damaged renal function suffer from significant changes in lipoprotein metabolism, which has a precise role in atherosclerotic pathogenesis. This is still controversial [35].

Uremia-Related Risk Factors

A known risk factor for the genesis of CV disease is $GFR<60ml/min/1.73m^2$. A further drop in GFR values, below $45ml/min/1.73m^2$, increases the risk of CV death. Potential factors tied to CKD and uremia, as well as the development of cardiovascular morbidity, includes inflammation, malnutrition, endothelial dysfunction, oxidative stress, vascular calcifications, vitamin D deficiency and hyperhomocysteinemia [36].

1. Inflammation

Inflammation, the effects of local inflammatory stimuli, such as oxidation products, end advanced glycosylation products and chronic infective processes modify blood vessels in the sense of atherosclerosis development. These changes benefit proatherogenic adhesion molecule production (e.g., ICAM-1 and VCAM-1), growth factor, as well as chemokine (such as IL-6 and TNF). Such inflammatory intermediates encourage synthesis of acute phase proteins, such as C-reactive protein (CRP), reduction of albumin synthesis in the liver of PD treated patients [31], which leads to endothelial dysfunction, which is usually defined as reduced vasodilatation capability, which again creates early atherosclerosis occurrence predisposition. However, the question, whether inflammation is a reflection of vascular damage, or actually supports factors that cause vascular injury, remains unanswered. The precise link between inflammation, endothelial dysfunction, oxidative stress, cardiovascular disease and mortality of PD patients remains unknown.

In a prospective study of PD patients, CRP level of >6mg/L was an independent predictive mark of possible myocardial infarction [37].

Aside from that, pro-inflammatory IL-6 mark is increased in ESRD patients, but is also an independent mortality predictor in patients on dialysis. Stompor and associates have shown that CRP, IL-6 and TNF levels are connected to increased thickness of the CCA in a group of PD patients monitored for over one year.

2. Endothelial Dysfunction

In PD patients, endothelial function is reduced, the same as in hemodialysis patients, most likely because of a reduced bioavailability of nitric oxide (NO) [38]. In a study conducted in 2009, flow mediated vasodilatation is significantly lower in PD patients than in the healthy population, which negatively correlates with inflammation markers, such as CRP or IL-6 [39]. There is evidence that suggests that the endogenic inhibitor of nitric oxide (NO), asymmetric dimethylarginine (ADMA), has a significant role in the origin and occurrence of cardiovascular diseases and mortality in PD patients. NO deficit and ADMA accumulation promote endothelial dysfunction, vasoconstriction and arterial thrombosis [40].

The remaining factors of endothelial dysfunction, such as soluble adhesive molecules are predictors of all causes of cardiovascular mortality in ESRD patients. The levels of vascular adhesive molecule-1 (VCAM-1) negatively correlate with LVH in PD patients.

3. Malnutrition and Protein-Energy Wasting

A marked connection between malnutrition, increased levels of CRP and atherosclerosis is well known, although the precise mechanisms of their synergistic effects on the organism are not known. This relationship was first described by Stenvinkel and associates in a study on CKD patients[41]. Patients with CKD levels >10mg/L have significantly lesser values of serum albumin and a higher prevalence of atherosclerosis than patients with a lower CKD level. The combination of malnutrition, inflammation and atherosclerosis presence has been described by Stenvinkel as MIA (Malnutrition Inflammation Atherosclerosis) syndrome. A 2008 study has shown that MIA syndrome is connected to increased mortality risks [42]. In a Korean study, comorbidity cardiovascular diseases were present in 78% of patients on PD with signs of malnutrition. These patients have a 3.3 times greater risk of mortality than patients suffering from malnutrition with no comorbidity conditions [43]. Taking malnutrition, protein deficits and inflammation into account, the recommendation for the description of this entity in CKD patients is protein-energy wasting (PEW) [44]. PEW is characterized by reduced protein and initiation energy accumulation. Several studies have shown that there are two types of malnutrition: the first is connected to poor food intake, and the second to inflammation and present comorbidity. Low levels of serum albumin can only be found in the second type of malnutrition, but the exact contribution of malnutrition or inflammation in the development of risk of CV mortality in PD patients remains uncertain [45].

A large number of studies have dealt in hypoalbuminemia, and the outcome of treating patients of PD. It has been determined that serum albumin levels below 40g/l are combined with a 4-20 times increased mortality. In addition, 45% of CAPD patients die during the first year of dialysis treatment in cases where albumin levels drop below 25 g/L. A CANUSA study has shown an 8% survival rate increase in cases of serum albumin growth of only 1%.

4. Oxidative Stress

Oxidative stress is defined as the damage of tissue which stems from the disturbed balance between excessive oxidation compound production and insufficient antioxidant defensive function. CKD patients have a deficiency in the antioxidant defensive mechanism (because of e.g., reduced vitamin levels, or hypoalbuminemia) and increased pro-oxidant compound activity (e.g., accumulation of solvent materials such as AGEs and β2-microglobulin). Oxidative stress leads to the production of free radicals, highly reactive compounds that can oxidize proteins lipids and nucleic acids. High concentrations of these molecules are present in CKD patients [46]. Oxidation products of proteins and oxidized DNA have been discovered in leukocytes with residual renal function. The underlying connection between increased levels of oxidation stress and the risk of cardiovascular death in ESRD patients is still unknown, even though the results of several prospective studies point to the conclusion that oxidation stress can be a risk factor in CV morbidity and mortality in ESRD patients [47, 48].

One of the more important toxins connected to the uremic environment and connected to oxidative stress and inflammation stage and the presence of inflammation biomarkers is beta$_2$ microglobulin. Increased levels of β_2-microglobulin in plasma are a known marker of chronic renal function failure, and are among the most important toxins tied to uremia. In PD patients, the level of β_2-microglobulin is primarily tied to amyloidosis.

In recent times it has been suggested that β_2-microglobulin could be a new biomarker of peripheral arterial disease and an independent predictor of aortic rigidity in the atherosclerotic process, in both the general population and ESRD patients [49]. Additionally, increased levels of β_2-microglobulin present a new marker for differentiating the levels of acute cardiac arrest creation risk in patients with creatinine levels $\leq 265\mu mol/L$ [50]. All of these results point to an important role of β_2-microglobulin in CV risk prediction on dialysis patients.

5. Calcification

Calcification of the arteries is an important risk factor for cardiovascular mortality in the general population. Hyperphosphatemia and increased Ca×P are known risk factors of CV diseases in both HD and PD patients [51]. These factors also contribute to general risk of vascular, and also valvular calcification, as well as calcifications in other tissues. Even though hyperphosphatemia is considered to be a relatively rare complication in PD patients, more and more evidence points to the fact that it is present in patients treated by peritoneal dialysis. The study on the adequacy of dialysis, and also the study of Wang and associates, showed that around 40% of patients on PD have serum phosphorus above targeted values of 1.78 mmol/L, values recommended by the Kidney Disease Outcomes Quality Initiative (KDOQI) [52].

One of the clinical consequences of hyperphosphatemia is the development of calcifications in blood vessels, valves and in other tissues. In hemodialysis patients the significance of calcified blood vessels in predicting cardiovascular mortality has been proven. Valvular calcifications are also a strong predictor of mortality in patients on PD [53]. The calcification of blood vessels in ESRD patients most commonly occurs in the intimal medial areas. Vascular calcifications caused by hyperphosphatemia usually occur in the blood vessel medial, connected to generalized arterial rigidity and increased after load of the cardiac muscle, which results in LVH and the reduction of the coronary reserve, with an increased risk of myocardial ischemia [54].

In PD patients, serum phosphorus and calcium phosphorus product (Ca × P) are the most important predictors of the advancement of carotid atherosclerosis and the development of CV diseases. However, the effects of hypocalcaemia (Vitamin D) and hyperparathyroidism, which are also included in the process of calcifications, are important [55]. The evidence that inflammation can also be involved in the process of calcification is numerous as well, which points to an important connection between inflammation and valvular calcifications. Wang and associates suggest that loss of RRF predisposes PD patients to valvular calcification, which is a consequence of high Ca × P product, and the presence of inflammation [56]. Inflammation, increased Ca × P, loss of RRF and valvular calcification in combination, synergistically act on the increased the risk of LVH development in PD patients. The process of calcification is, therefore, under the influence of numerous factors, those which favor calcium deposition, and others, such as GLA protein and fetuin-a, which act oppositely.

Fibroblast growth factor-23 (FGF-23) is a hormone that is involved in regulating phosphorus levels and vitamin D metabolism [57]. The level of this hormone grows in the early stages of CRF and causes the loss of phosphorus by inhibiting the sodium-dependent phosphate cotransporter, NPC tip IIa in proximal renal tubule. It suffocates the expression of renal CIP27B1 (cytochrome P450, family 27, subfamily B, polypeptide 1), which leads to calcitriol synthesis disorders. FGF-23 also controls the mineralization of bones independently of phosphate homeostasis [58]. In animal tests, as well as in studies on humans, it has been noted that its reduced activity is connected to vascular soft tissue calcifications [59].

6. Hyperparathyroidism

In ESRD patients, the ability of the diseased kidney to produce 1.25-dihydroxycalciferol is reduced, which significantly contributes to the development of osteodystrophy, secondary hyperparathyroidism and the disturbed metabolism of divalent ions. Parathormone is considered a potent uremic toxin that harmfully affects myocardial cells. The improvement of left ventricular dysfunction after parathyroidectomy in uremic patients with increased PTH, points to a connection between left ventricular function and hyperparathyroidism. All this confirms the assumption about the role of parathormone as a risk factor in the development of uremic cardiomyopathy.

Significant research results point to the conclusion that a small level of vitamin D is connected to cardiovascular disease in the general population, and that a greater concentration of that vitamin can have a positive influence on survival. Similar results were discovered in pre-dialysis patients. Wang and associates have determined that low concentrations of serum 25-hydroxyvitamin Din PD patients are connected to increased risk of fatal or non-fatal cardiovascular incidents. It seems that the effects of vitamin D on the cardiovascular system are connected to residual renal function, LVH and cardiac dysfunction [60].

7. Hyperhomocysteinemia

High levels of homocysteine are present in 90% of CKD patients, which can contribute to early onset atherosclerosis and cardiovascular diseases [61]. Results of clinical trials, in which the relation between Hyperhomocysteinemia and cardiovascular diseases that are researched are contradictory, so that there exists a hypothesis of so called reverse epidemiology, that is, that low levels of homocysteine are connected with a poor prognosis [62]. Still, in multiple studies, independent function of homocysteine on the origin of cardiovascular diseases in dialysis patients has been determined [63]. Homocysteine has shown itself to be an important predictor in the origin and development of carotid atherosclerosis in PD patients [64].

8. Insulin Resistance

Available data shows that insulin resistance (IR) is present in CKD patients starting from the early stages of renal failure. The potential of IR to promote blood vessel damage, regardless of the coexistence of other vascular risk factors, is large [65]. In several studies, the role of IR in patients on PD was analyzed, and a connection between IR and a disturbed fatty acid metabolism has been discovered, which further contributed to left ventricular dysfunction. Also, more and more evidence points to the fact that the application of ACE inhibitors can modulate IR. In PD, insulin resistance of the tissue can be worsened by the intake of glucose through dialysis solutions. However, these studies are controversial as well: in patients on cycler PD, IR is greater than HD patients, while in CAPD patients, IR is normalized, similar to hemodialysis patients. By using icodextrin dialysis solutions, insulin levels in serum could potentially be reduced, and insulin sensitivity increased [66].

9. Anemia

Anemia, as a basic marking of ESRD, is a significant factor connected to the development of uremic cardiomyopathy, cardiac failure, and mortality. The effects of anemia to the cardiovascular system are connected to hemodynamic changes and the increase of minute volume, as a compensatory response to reduced oxygen transport [67]. These effects of anemia contribute to the development of LV dilation, and compensatory LVH, which can consequently lead to cardiac failure with a fatal outcome.

On the other hand, studies on subjects suffering from CKD (Treat, Choir and Create) have shown that hemoglobin correction to normal levels did not improve the survival rate. However, in a study of 1265 HD patients, with verifiable cardiac failure or ischemic heart disease, there was a greater mortality and non-fatal myocardial infarction rate in patients who had hematocrite of greater values, in relation to subjects with lower hematocrit levels. Moreover, the application of iron in anemia therapy increased oxidative stress, and thus contributed to increased cardiovascular mortality risk in ESRD patients [68].

HD and PD are significantly different, and their differences can affect the occurrence of anemia, the diagnosis and control of anemia. Despite the fact that PD is considered an equivalent alternative to HD, and is universally applied, most data that studied the commonality of anemia related factors and clinical guidelines for treatment stem from studies performed on the HD population [69].

Risk Factors Related to Peritoneal Dialysis

All risk factors of the origin of CV diseases and mortality risk, present in ESRD patients, are found in PD patients. However, key differences in risk factor of CV diseases exist between PD and ESRD patients.

The intake of dialysis solution into the peritoneal cavity not only causes increased intraperitoneal pressure, but also causes an increase in systemic blood flow due to the increase of general peripheral resistance [70]. Dialysis influent also leads to an increase in the levels of atrial natriuretic peptide (ANP) in plasma, but it is not known whether these acute changes in ANP concentration can be considered a risk factor for cardiovascular diseases [70].

Conventional solutions for PD contain extremely high concentrations of glucose (>200 mmol/L), as well as glucose degradation products (GDPs), which are produced during the sterilization of the solution with heat. Waste products of glucose mainly consist of aldehydes and dicarbonyl compounds, and lactates, which are used as stabilizers in conventional solutions. On average, 65% of total glucose in one dialysis bag is absorbed during 4 hours of presence of dialysate in the peritoneal cavity, regardless of the original concentration of glucose in the dialysate [70]. In extreme situations, this process can lead to further carbohydrate encumbrance, in excess of 500 grams/day. This excess of carbohydrates can lead to the development of obesity, insulin resistance and atherogenic lipid profile [71].

1. Dialysis Solutions and Advanced Glycation End-Products

Constant exposure to extremely high concentrations of glucose in dialysate leads to the production of advanced glycation end-products (AGEs) in the peritoneal tissue. The contribution of AGEs in the origin of arterial rigidity cannot be understated, especially when glucose absorption through the peritoneum leads to hyperglycemia. Concentrations of AGEs in plasma are increased in PD patients compared to healthy persons, while concentrations of AGEs do not significantly differ in HD and PD patients [70].

The application of biocompatible dialysis solutions reduces the concentration of end-products of glucose, though the clinical relevance to the applications of such solutions remains unknown in relation to their effect on cardiovascular mortality of PD patients [72]. The Euro-Balance Trial gave a recommendation that the preservation of RRF is better and more efficient in using a biocompatible solution in relation to conventional ones [73]. However, such a position has not been confirmed by randomized, controlled studies in PD patients. The use of biocompatible dialysis solution will likely lead to a direct reduction of cardiovascular risk factors by reducing peritoneal neoangiogenesis, thus reducing the risk of ultrafiltration deficit, and potentially protecting the system from the origin of encapsulating peritoneal sclerosis.

2. Residual Renal Function (RRF)

Residual renal function is important to PD patients because it contributes to total daily clearance of 20% or more [74]. It is thought that a PD patient has preserved RRF if his clearance of creatinine is greater than 1.5 ml/min.

In PD patients, RRF is connected to all causes of mortality, and so it is connected with the risk of cardiovascular death [75]. The vital role of RRF in the survival of PD patients was determined in large prospective studies, such as the CANUSA and ADEMEX studies. Prospective cohort reanalysis of the CANUSA study, on a group of 601 PD patients, clearly determined that patient survival is connected with RRF and weekly diuresis (5L per week/m^2). GFR increase corresponds to a 12% reduction in relative risk of mortality [76].

In the ADEMEX study, by a prospective, randomized examination of 965 PD patients with a weekly diuresis of 10L/m^2, a relative mortality risk drop of 11% was noted [77]. These results were also confirmed by the NECOSAD study, where the rate of reduction of RRF was a stronger predictor of mortality and technical insufficiency of long term PD treatment, in relation to basic RRF [78]. Wang and associates have proven the connection between RRF and LVH in PD diabetic patients [79].

3. Volume Overload and Ultrafiltration Insufficiency

Ultrafiltration insufficiency occurs in around a third of PD patients, and can lead to arterial hypertension and volume encumbrance. Volume overload promoted the development of LVH and leads to increased serum concentrations of natriuretic peptide, because of their increased myocardial production. These peptides are used as a prognostic marker for the general mortality of ESRD patients [80]. High concentrations of ANP in plasma and B-type natriuretic peptide (BNP) in PD patients are connected to approximately eight times greater mortality risk in comparison with patients with low concentrations of these peptides [81].

The connection between the lack of peritoneal ultrafiltration and mortality has been proven in anuric patients. When fluid intake is not adjusted to peritoneal ultrafiltration, the patient will develop volume overload, which increases the risk of cardiovascular diseases [82].

4. Genetic and Epigenetic Factors

Genetic factors can influence the appearance and frequency of vascular complications in PD patients. Thus, polymorphism of a single nucleotide in the IL-6 gene is connected to increased levels of IL-6 in plasma, and comorbidity in HD patients [83], greater diastolic pressure values and left ventricular mass [84]. Polymorphism of the enzyme, which transforms angiotensin I to angiotensin II, can determine the degree of the function of recombined human erythropoietin in PD patients, which presents a significant prescreening for the assessment of erythropoietin resistance.

Polymorphism on the humane receptor of Vitamin D is combined with an increased risk of the development of hypercalcemia, modulation of NO activity via the polymorphism of endothelial NOS, as well as functionally relevant polymorphism of the IL-6, which together can have a significant effect on basic peritoneal permeability [85]. In the future, research in this field could enable a more precise approach to the identification of risk groups of patients treated by PD, and the development of personalized treatment strategies.

A new approach in the research of atherosclerosis focuses on the role of epigenetics, which change studies in gene expression that are not coded in the DNA sequence itself, but are instead a consequence of post-translatory changes in the DNA protein. These epigenetic changes can be lost in several sequential cellular generations. Changes of the genome methylation of DNA have important regulatory functions in normal and pathological cellular processes. A persistent inflammatory reaction is most likely connected to DNA hypermethylation [86]. Further research is necessary to determine whether epigenetic DNA changes are connected to accelerated atherosclerosis in uremia.

2. Aims

- To evaluate functional-morphological characteristics of the left ventricle and morphological characteristics of carotid arteries in ESRD patients at the start and after 18 months of treatment with continuous ambulatory peritoneal dialysis.
- To examine the presence of traditional and uremia-related risk factors of cardiovascular disease, as well as those connected with peritoneal dialysis during the monitoring period.
- To evaluate the relative significance of dialysis efficiency, and transport characteristics of the peritoneum, for cardiovascular morbidity in patients on PD.
- To estimate the ratio of individual risk factors in the origin of cardiovascular diseases in peritoneal dialysis patients, through morphological-functional changes of the left ventricle, and morphological changes on carotid arteries in patients at the beginning and after 18 months of PD treatment.

3. METHODS

Patients

This prospective longitudinal study included 50 ESRD that were observed for 18 months after the commencement of continuous ambulatory PD (CAPD) treatment. Other than excluding patients with congenital or valvular heart disease, cerebral vascular diseases, patients with underlying active inflammatory disease such as systemic lupus erythematosus, malignancy, as well as patients previously treated with hemodialysis, all non-anuric CAPD patients were included in the study. All examined patients underwent four to five dialysis changes with 2 L of dialysis solution. Double-chamber bag Stay-Safe® Balance system (Fresenius Medical Care, Germany) was available for all, including patients. This system utilizes a lactate-buffered PD solution in a two-compartment bag offered in the Stay-Safe® disconnect system. The formation of glucose degradation product (GDP) is greatly reduced by separating the glucose component of the solution (kept at very low pH) from the lactate component of the solution (kept at alkaline pH) during sterilization and storage. Immediately before infusion, the seam between the two chambers is opened, and the contents are mixed. The ready-to-use solution has a near-physiological pH, and a greatly reduced amount of GDP.

At the moment of the start trial, all observed patients were without clinical manifestation of heart failure.

The base laboratory assessment included measurement of brain-natriuretic peptide (BNP) as well as serum endothelin-1 (ET-1) and nitric oxide (NO) concentration. The measurement of serum concentration of ET-1 (pg/mL) was done by the ELISA method (Enzyme immunoassay for the quantitative determination of human endothelin (1–21) in serum, kit Biomedica Medizinprodukte GmbH & Co KG, Wien). For the determination of concentration of NO in the serum, R&D System Total Nitric Oxide kit was utilized, while the concentration of NO was expressed in µmol/L. Blood samples for the determination of concentration of NO and ET-1 were analyzed at the Institute for Biochemistry of the Clinical Hospital *Sestre milosrdnice* in Zagreb, Croatia.

In all patients, any therapy that can influence the values of monitored laboratory parameters (nitrites, captopril, NSAIDs, heparin, beta2 agonists)were excluded 24 h before taking blood samples for determination of concentration of ET-1 and NO. The study was conducted 2 h after an early morning dialysis change. All records of patients were protected, whereas the study was conducted with the approval of the local Ethics Committee and respect for the rules of ethic principles in medical research. All patients gave their informed consent for participation in the study.

Echocardiographic Assessment

In all patients echocardiographic parameters were evaluated at the very beginning of dialysis treatment and after 18 months. Echocardiographic assessment was conducted using the "Toshiba 270 SSA" device, equipped with the 3.75MHz frequency sector sonde. All patients were examined with the method of conventional M-mode and two-dimensional echocardiography. The measurement performed by two cardiologists, who were not acquainted with the clinical status of the patients, according to the recommendations of the American Society of Echocardiography. The LV mass was calculated according to the formula of Penn Convention [87], while the left ventricular mass index (LVMi) was calculated with the division of the left ventricular mass (LVM) with the body surface area. LVH is defined as the LVMi > 131 g/m^2 for males and >00 g/m^2 for females. The systolic function of the LV was assessed by the measurement of ejection fraction (EF). The systolic weakness of LV is defined as EF < 50%. The diastolic function of LV is assessed by determination of the maximum velocity of the early (E) and late (A) phase of ventricular filling and the calculation of the E/A ratio. The diastolic dysfunction of LV is defined as $E/A \leq 1$.

Parameters of Peritoneal Dialysis

The indices of dialysis adequacy were measured after six and eighteen months after the patient started PD. Adequacy of dialysis (Kt/Vurea) was calculated from total weekly removed urea mass by daily volume of dialysate and urine (Kt) and divided with urea distribution volume (V). The distribution volume of urea was calculated using the Watson equation [88].

Residual renal function was estimated as the mean of renal creatinine and renal urea clearance (mL/min) at baseline and at the end of the study period. A simplified peritoneal equilibration test was performed using a 4.25% glucose-based solution to obtain the dialysate to plasma creatinine concentration ratio at 4 hours of dwell (D/P [Cr]). Patients were categorized as high, high-average, and low-average transporters according to criteria of Chung and colleagues [88].

Ultrasound Examination of the Carotid Arteries

The severity of carotid artery atherosclerosis was evaluated using the mean common carotid artery (CA) intima-media thickness (mean IMT) and plaque score (PS). Carotid ultrasonography was used to evaluate the mean IMT and the PS. High-resolution B mode, color Doppler, and pulse Doppler ultrasonography of both carotid arteries were performed with an ultrasound scanner (Wall-Track system: W-T, Maastricht, the Netherlands) equipped with a 7.5-MHZ linear array transducer by the same experienced angiologist. Measurement was done by the angiologist who was not familiar with the clinical status of the study patients. Patients were examined in the supine position with the head tilted backwards. After the carotid arteries were located by transverse scans, the probe was rotated 90° to obtain and record a longitudinal image of the anterior and posterior walls. The high-resolution images of the far wall of the bilateral CA, internal carotid arteries (ICA), and carotid bulbs were examined according to recommendations of the American Society of Echocardiography Carotid Intima Media Thickness Task Force [89]. The IMT was defined as the distance between the leading edge of the lumen-intima echo and the leading edge of the media-adventitia echo. At least three measurements were taken over a 1-cm length of the far wall of each CA segment, and these measurements were averaged on both sides to obtain the mean IMT. The PS was calculated by adding the maximal thickness in millimetres of plaques in each segment on both sides (A + B + C + thickness of the contralateral carotid artery plaques). The length of individual plaques was not considered in determining the PS.

The presence of atherosclerosis in CCA is estimated as recommended by the Mannheim consensus about atherosclerosis [89]:

(1) Without atherosclerosis (AS 0): IMT less than 80% of the reference interval (RI), adjusted by age and gender. RI values were obtained from previously published studies of monitoring, using the same ultrasound procedures.

(2) Mild atherosclerosis (AS 1): IMT > 80% RI.

(3) Moderate atherosclerosis (AS 2): the presence of carotid plaque, with no significant stenosis (PSV < 125 cm/s)

(4) Severe atherosclerosis (AS 3): the presence of carotid plaque with threatening stenosis (PSV > 125 cm/s).

Statistical Analysis

All statistical calculations were performed with the SPSS 16 software (version 16.0, SPSS Inc., Chicago, IL). Each value was expressed as the mean±SD or as median and interquartile range where appropriate. Significant changes in the variables from baseline to 18 months after PD treatment were tested by paired t-test for the variables that followed normal distribution or by the Wilcoxon signed-rank test for the variables that had skewed distribution. The difference between the two groups was analyzed by the Mann–Whitney test. A multiple regression analysis was applied to examine the relationship between LV remodeling parameters and a set of clinical and laboratory parameters. Since ET-1, NO, C-reactive protein (CRP), B-type natriuretic peptide (BNP), and age were non-normally distributed in this study, we normalized these data by log transformation before entering a stepwise multiple regression. The significant independent variables were ordered according to their standardized effect, defined as regression coefficient/standard error of the regression (b). P values <0.05 were considered statistically significant.

4. RESULTS

The most common renal disease, which leads to end stage renal function failure, is diabetic nephropathy (48%), followed by chronic pyelonephritis (18%).Nephroangiosclerosis and chronic glomerulonephritis are equally represented as causes in ESRD subjects (14%) (Table 1).

Blood pressure is statistically significantly lower after 18 months of peritoneal dialysis treatment compared to basal values. Statistically significant differences in BMI values have not been found. Lipid values in patient serum are statistically significantly lower after 18 months of PD, while HDL cholesterol values are significantly increased at the end follow-up (Table 2).

The results of peritoneal dialysis effects on uremic parameters are displayed in Table 3. Treatment by peritoneal dialysis results in a significant drip of nitrogen matter in blood (p < 0.001), with a simultaneous significant increase of RRF (p < 0.001) and a significant increase of average PCR values as the predictor of nutrition status (p < 0.001).

Table 1. Cause of ESRD and characteristics of study subjects

Diabetic nephropathy	24 (48%)
Hypertensive nephrosclerosis	7 (14%)
Pyelonephritis	9 (18%)
Glomerulonephritis	7 (14%)
Reflux nephropathy	2 (4%)
Unknown	1 (2%)
Age (y)	60.5 (26-76)
Male	25 (50%)
Diabetes mellitus tip 2	26 (52%)
Smoker (yes)	18 (45%)

Data are expressed as number(percentage).

Table 2. Traditional risk factors in ESRD and PD patients

	Baseline	12 months on PD	18 months on PD	p
SBP(mmHg)	147.4 ± 20.1	134.2 ± 14.4	129.4 ± 11.5	<0.001
DBP (mmHg)	89.2 ± 12.6	79.4 ± 9.8	78.4 ± 7.9	<0.001
MBP (mmHg)	109.2 ± 15.1	96.5 ± 12.0	95.4 ± 8.2	<0.001
BMI (kg/m^2)	25.9 ± 3.7	25.8 ± 2.6	25.7 ± 2.2	NS
Cholesterol (mmol/L)	6.5 ± 1.6	5.9 ± 1.2	5.5 ± 1.3	<0.001
Triglyceride (mmol/L)	2.4 ± 1.3	1.7 ± 0.4	2.0 ± 2.5	<0.001
HDL (mmol/L)	1.0 ± 0.3	1.3 ± 0.3	1.4 ± 0.3	<0.001
LDL (mmol/L)	4.7 ± 1.4	3.8 ± 0.8	3.6 ± 0.8	<0.001
Lp(a) (g/L)	0.5 ± 0.2	0.3 ± 0.2	0.3 ± 0.1	<0.001
Apo B (g/L)	1.3 ± 0.4	1.2 ± 0.3	1.2 ± 0.3	<0.001
Apo A I (g/L)	1.4 ± 0.4	1.9 ± 0.3	1.8 ± 0.3	<0.001

Note: SBP, systolic blood pressure; DBP, diastolic BP; MBP, mean BP; BMI, body mass index; HDL, high-density lipoprotein; LDL, low-density lipoprotein; Lp(a), lipoprotein(a); Apo B, apolipoprotein B; Apo A, apolipoprotein A I.

Data are expressed as mean ± SD.

After 18 months of CAPD treatment, a significant decrease of average beta 2-microglobulin, CaxP, CRP and fibrinogen was observed in patients in relation to the same values observed immediately before dialysis treatment. The levels of parathyroid hormone did not significantly change at the end of the study in relation to baseline.

Median BNP, troponin and tHcy values are significantly lower after 12 and 18 months of peritoneal dialysis treatment in relation to basal values before dialysis treatment.

Table 3. Clinical, biochemical and dialytic parameters of the groups of PD patients during the monitoring period

	Baseline	After 18 months on PD	p
Diuresis (mL/24h)	545.6 ± 378.5	584.8 ±489.7	NS
RRF (ml/min)	5.5 ± 3.8	7.0 ± 5.0	<0.001
Urea (mmol/L)	25.7 ± 6.7	17.5 ± 2.5	<0.001
Creatinine (mmol/L)	912.3 ± 223.3	733.9 ± 131.0	<0.001
CRP (mg/L)	11.1 (6.1-16.4)	4.5 (2.8-7.7)	<0.001
Fibrinogen (g/L)	6.2 ± 1.9	4.4 ± 1.3	<0.001
Ca (mmol/L)	2.2 ± 0.2	2.3 ± 0.1	NS
P (mmol/L)	1.8 ± 0.3	1.6 ± 0.2	<0.001
CaxP	3.9 ± 0.6	3.6 ± 0.5	<0.001
PTH (pg/ml)	225.5(97.8-387)	200.0 (100.0-410)	NS
PCRg/kg/24h	0.98 ± 0.13	1.11 ± 0.1	<0.001
β_2 microglobulin (μg/mL)	7.0 (2.9-11.2)	4.2 (2.3-9.7)	<0.001
Hb (g/L)	101.9 ± 10.3	118.6 ± 11.1	<0.001
Albumin (g/L)	30.9 ± 2.6	31.5 ± 2.0	<0.01
Proteinuria (g/24h)	0.79 ± 0.41	0,70 ± 0.39	0.05

Note: RRF, residual renal function; CRP, C-reactive protein; Ca, calcium; P, phosphorus; PTH, parathyroid hormone; PCR, protein catabolic rate; Hb, hemoglobin, NS, non significant. Data are expressed as mean±SD, or median(range).

Table 4. Biomarkers of cardiovascular remodeling

BNP (pg/mL)	183.9 (89.8-432.5)	90.3 (67.8-154.3)	69.6 (50.2-98.8)	<0.001
Troponin (ng/mL)	0.022 (0.001-0.12)	0.01 (0.00-0.041)	0.001 (0.0-0.01)	<0.001
tHcy (μmol/L)	25.2 (20.2-30.1)	21.0 (16.7-23.4)	18.0 (14.0-20.9)	<0.001

Note: BNP, B-type natriuretic peptide, tHcy, total homocysteine. Data are expressed as median (range).

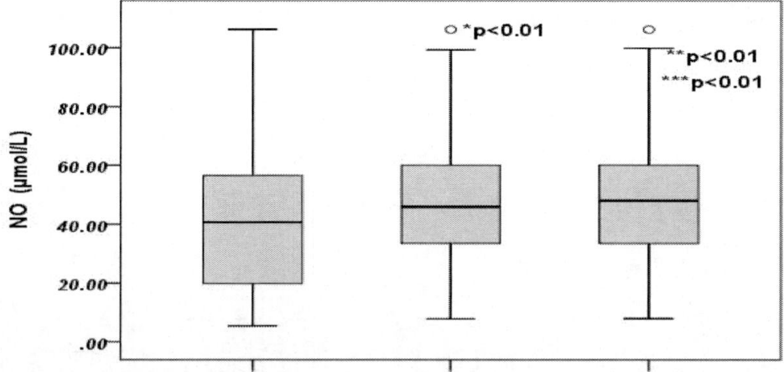

Baseline12 months on PD18 months on PD

Data are expressed as mean±SD, or median(range).

*Significant difference between 12 months on PD and baseline.

**Significant difference between 12 and 18 months on PD

*** Significant difference between 18 months on PD and baseline

Figure 1. Nitric oxide at baseline and after18 months on peritoneal dialysis.

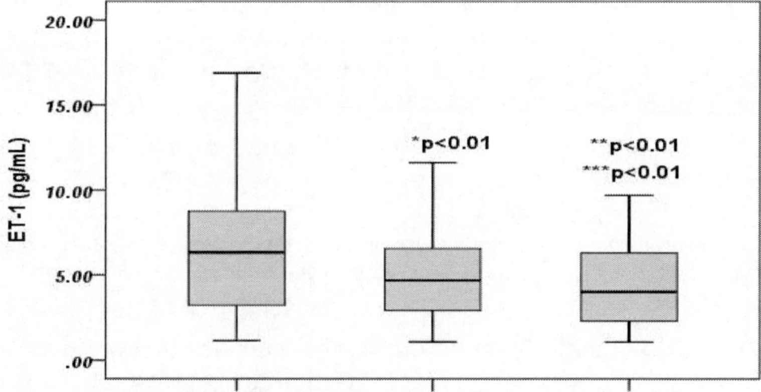

Baseline 12 months on PD18 months on PD

Data are expressed as mean±SD, or median(range).

*Significant difference between 12 months on PD and baseline.

**Significant difference between 12 and 18 months on PD

*** Significant difference between 18 months on PD and baseline

Figure 2. Endothelin-1 at baseline and after 18 months on peritoneal dialysis.

Table 5. Echocardiographic analysis of monitored PD patients

	Baseline n=50	18 months PD n=50	p
EF (%)	50.1 ±9.4	56.9 ± 10.0	0.002
E/A ratio	1.0 ± 0.1	1.1 ± 0.1	<0.05
LVEDD (mm)	52.9 ± 3.6	49.6 ± 6.5	<0.001
LVDS (mm)	35.0 ± 3.5	34.3 ± 3.9	0.05
LVMi (g/m^2)	162.2 ± 38.1	140.2 ± 37.8	<0.001
LVM (gr)	280.7 ± 43.2	243.8 ± 40.8	<0.001
LVV (mL/m^2)	90.2 ± 24.5	83.8 ± 21.7	<0.001
LAD (mm)	43.3 ± 5.7	40.5 ± 6.7	<0.05
FS (%)	28.8 ± 5.1	30.8 ± 4.1	<0.001

Note: EF, ejection fraction; LVEDD, left ventricular end. diastolic diameter; LVDS, left ventricular systolic diameter, LVMI- LV mass index; LVM, LV mass; LVV, LV volume; LAD, left atrium diameter; FS, fractional shortening.

Median value of NO in patient serum on PD was basally 40.72 (19.4-56, 7) μmol/L and is statistically significantly greater after 12 months (45.95 (33.5-60.0) μmol/L and 18 months (48.0 (32.8-60.4) μmol/L) of peritoneal dialysis treatment in relation to basal values ($p < 0.0001$) (Figure 1).

Median ET-1 values after 18 months of CAPD treatment (4.0 (2.27 - 6.3) pg/ml) are statistically significantly lower in relation to values after 12 months (4.68 (2.9-6.6) pg/ml and basal values (6.32 (3.2-8.8) pg/ml) ($p < 0.001$) (Figure 2).

A statistically significant reduction of left ventricular mass index in the observed population of subjects was registered after 18 months on PD treatment in relation to basal results. (140.2 ± 37.8 vs. 162.2 ± 38.1 g/m²; $p < 0.001$).

A statistically significant improvement of ejection fraction was discovered after 18 months of CAPD treatment, in relation to basal values (50.1% vs. 56.9%;$p < 0.002$), as well as significant repair of diastolic function estimated by the E/A ratio (1.1 ± 0.1. vs. 1.0 ± 0.1; <0.05). A significantly larger percentage of patients with regular left ventricular function was observed after 18 months on PD in relation to ESRD patients (64% vs. 20%) ($p < 0.001$).

Left ventricular hypertrophy was found in 78% of patients before the beginning of peritoneal dialysis treatment. A year and a half after dialysis treatment a significantly lessened number of LVH patients was observed, which was found in 60% of treated patients ($p = 0.004$). Concentric LVH was found in 61.5% of patients with pre-treatment.

A similar amount of patients with concentric LVH was (63.3%) was discovered after 18 months of PD treatment (Table 13).

Before the start of dialysis treatment in LVH patients, the average values of systolic and diastolic blood pressure were statistically significantly greater than in patients not suffering from LVH (p < 0.01), as well as average values of median arterial blood pressure (p < 0.03). However after 18 months on peritoneal dialysis treatment values of both systolic and diastolic pressure both dropped significantly, as well as values of median arterial blood pressure, in relation to basal values, in both patient groups, with a stronger, more pronounced drop in the LVH patient group (SBP 134.3 ± 11,7 vs. 152.8 ± 19.1 mmHg; DBP 80.3 ± 8.5 vs. 92.1 ± 12.0 mmHg; MBP 98.3 ± 8.4 vs. 111.8 ± 13.7 mmHg) (Table 7).

In LVH patients, the average values of serum lipids were statistically significantly greater than in patients without LVH, basally as well as after 18 months of monitoring. After 18 months on PD, there was a significant reduction in all fractions of serum lipids in relation to basal values.

Table 6. Left ventricular structure in PD patients during 18 month period

		Baseline	12 months PD	18 months PD	p
Without LVH		11 (22.0%)	16 (32.0%)	20 (40%)	0.004*
LVH		39 (78.0%)	34 (68.0%)	30 (60%)	
LVH	Concentric	24 (61.5%)	24 (70.6%)	19 (63.3%)	NS*
	Eccentric	15 (38.5%)	10 (29.4%)	11 (36.7%)	

Note: LVH, left ventricular hypertrophy; NS-non significant.

Table 7. Traditional risk factors and left ventricular modification

Baseline				18 months on PD		
	Normal LV (n=11)	LVH (n=39)	p	Normal LV(n=20)	LVH (n=30)	p
SBP (mmHg)	128.2 ± 8.7	152.8 ± 19.1	<0.01	122.0 ± 6.2	134.3 ± 11.7**	<0.01
DBP (mmHg)	79.1 ± 9.4	92.1 ± 12.0	<0.01	75.5 ± 6.1	80.3 ± 8.5**	0.04
MBP (mmHg)	100.0 ± 16.9	111.8 ± 13.7	0.03	91.0 ± 5.4	98.3 ± 8.4**	<0.01
BMI (kg/m^2)	23.9 ± 3.4	26.5 ± 3.6	NS	24.6 ± 2.2	26.4 ± 1.9	<0.01
Cholesterol (mmol/L)	5.7 ± 1.9	6.7 ± 1.5	0.046	4.5 ± 0.6	6.1 ± 1.3**	<0.01

Table 7. (Continued)

Baseline				18 months on PD		
	Normal LV (n=11)	LVH (n=39)	p	Normal LV(n=20)	LVH (n=30)	p
Triglyceride (mmol/L)	2.0 ± 1.5	2.5 ± 1.2	NS	1.4 ± 0.4	2.4 ± 3.1**	<0.01
HDL (mmol/L)	1.4 ± 0.3	1.0 ± 0.2	<0.01	1.6 ± 0.2*	1.2 ± 0.2**	<0.01
LDL (mmol/L)	3.8 ± 1.9	5.0 ± 1.2	<0.01	2.9 ± 0.7	4.1 ± 0.5**	<0.01
Lp(a) (g/L)	0.3 ± 0.1	0.5 ± 0.2	<0.01	0.2 ± 0.1*	0.3 ± 0.1**	<0.01
Apo B (g/L)	1.0 ± 0.4	1.4 ± 0.3	<0.01	1.1 ± 0.3	1.3 ± 0.3**	<0.01
Apo A I(g/L)	1.3 ± 0.4	1.4 ± 0.4	NS	1.6 ± 0.3*	2.0 ± 0.3**	<0.01

*Significant difference between at baseline and after 18 months on PD in the same group.
** Significant difference between at baseline and after 18 months on PD in the same group.

The average values of creatinin and urea were significantly greater in LVH patients in relation to patients without LVH, at the beginning of dialysis treatment, and after an 18 month period of peritoneal dialysis treatment ($p<0.01$), but with a significant reduction of their levels in both patient groups during monitoring period (Table 8).

Table 8. Uremia-related risk factors and left ventricular modification

	Baseline			18 months PD		
	Normal LV (n=11)	LVH (n=39)	p	Normal LV (n=20)	LVH (n=30)	p
Urea (mmol/L)	21.1 ±6.3	27.0±6.3	<0.01	15.8±2.9*	18.6±1.3**	<0.01
Creatinine (mmol/L)	763.9±289.3	954.2±184	0.04	655.1±128	786.4±104	<0.01
ß$_2$microgl. (μg/mL)	2.2±0.2	11.4±8.8	<0.01	3.9±4.4	10.9±11.3	<0.01
Ca (mmol/L)	2.3±0.1	2.2±.2	NS	2.3±0.1	2.3±0.1	NS
P (mmol/L)	1.5±0.2	1.8±0.3	<0.01	1.4±0.2	1.7±0.2**	<0.01
CaxP	3.3±0.6	4.0±.5	<0.01	3.3±0.5	3.8±0.5**	<0.01
PTH (pg/mL)	173.6±133.0	290.0±210	NS	189.4±209	327.4±214.7	<0.01
CRP (mg/L)	5.7±3.5	13.9±8.4	<0.01	2.6±1.3*	6.4±2.9**	<0.01
Fibrinogen (g/L)	4.3±1.9	6.7±1.5	<0.01	3.5±0.8	5.0±1.2**	<0.01
Hb (g/L)	108.8±10.7	99.9±9.4	<0.01	126.7±7.3*	113.3±10**	<0.01
Albumin (g/L)	34.9±4.3	29.5±3.8	NS	33.1±1.7*	30.4±1.4	<0.01
Proteinuria (g/day)	0.79±0.93	1.24±1.03	<0.05	0.72±0.62*	0.9±0.83**	<0.05

*Significant difference between without LVH at baseline and after 18 months on PD.
**Significant difference between with LVH at baseline and after 18 months on PD.

The average values of Beta 2-microglobulin, Caxp product, CRP, and fibrinogen were statistically significantly greater in patients with LVH ($p < 0.01$). In the LVH patient group a significantly larger phosphate average value in serum was determined, in relation to patients without LVH ($p < 0.01$)m before dialysis treatment, as well as after 18 months of dialysis treatment. Average PTH values in plasma were significantly greater in LVH patients, compared to the group with no LVH (Table 8).

A marked drop in average values of CaxP, CRP, and fibrinogen was noted after 18 months of CAPD treatment in relation to values before treatment with LVH and without LVH ($p < 0.01$). Average hemoglobin values were significantly smaller in LVH patients compared to the group without LVH, before ($p < 0.01$) and after 18 months of CAPD treatment ($p < 0.01$). The loss of protein through urine significantly differed between the two groups at the beginning and the end of the monitoring period (<0.05).

Table 9. Peritoneal dialysis specific risk factors and left ventricular modification

		Baseline			After 18 months on PD		
		Normal LV (n=11)	Normal LV (n=39)	p	Normal LV (n=20)	LVH (n=30)	p
Kt/V	<1.7	0	4(10.3%)		0	1 (3.3%)	
	1.7-2.0	0	21(53.8%)	<0.01	1 (5.0%)	18(60.0%)	<0.01
	>2.0	11(100%)	14(35.9%)		19(95.0%)	11(36.7%)	
PCR g/kg/24h		1.1±0.1	1.0±0.1	<0.01	1.2±0.1	1.1±0.1	<0.01
Protein loss (PD effluent)(g)		6.2±2.1	6.1±1.9	NS	6.55±1.1	5.9±1.7	0.05
Diuresis (ml/d)		750.0±463.1	487.9±335.9	NS	897.5±555.7	376.3±300.7	<0.01
RRF (ml/min)		7.2±4.2	5.0±3.5	NS	9.8±5.4	5.1±3.8	<0,01
Low-average transporters (T) n(%)		11(100%)	23(59%)	<0.01	20 (100%)	1 (53.3%)	<0.01
High-average T n (%)		0	9(23.1%)		0	9 (30.0%)	
High T n (%)		0	7(17.9%)		0	5 (16.7%)	

Residual renal function did not significantly differ between the two patient groups in relation to LVH presence. However in patients with echographically sound LV results, after 18 months of CAPD treatment, average RRF values were statistically significantly greater than in relation to LVH patients. ($p< 0.01$) It was determined that all patients without LVH had an estimated adequacy of dialysis treatment of Kt/V > 2.0, while in 53.8% of LVH patients in the first 6 months of treatment the value of Kt/V was 1.7-2, which was statistically significant (p < 0.01). Also, after 18 months of CAPD treatment in 60% of LVH patients Kt/V values were 1.7 - 2.0, while 95% of patients without LVH had a Kt/V value of >2.0, which was also statistically significant (p < 0.01). The loss of protein through dialysis effluent did not statistically differ between observed groups at the beginning of the study, but after 18 months of PD treatment the loss of protein through dialysate was significantly greater in the LVH group (0.05). Average PCR values were significantly lower in LVH patients in relation to patients without LVH (Table 9).

Median values of BNP, troponin, NO and ET-1 markers were significantly higher in LVH patients at the beginning of PD treatment, but also after 12 and 18 months of PD treatment, in relation to patients with no LVH. A significant drop in median values of BNP, troponin and homocysteine was noted in the LVH patient group 18 months after the beginning of PD treatment in relation to basal values. Median values of NO and ET-1 changed significantly during the monitoring period, both in LVH and non-LVH patients (Table 10).

Table 10. Biomarkers of cardiovascular remodeling during follow-up

	Baseline			After 18 months PD		
	Normal LV(n=11)	LVH (n=39)	p	Normal LV (n=20)	LVH (n=30)	p
BNP (pg/mL)	58.3 (50-197.9)	266.4 (117.8-528.8)	0.017	53.0 (30.2-77.0)	79.1 (66.9-112.4)**	<0.001
Troponin (ng/mL)	0.00	0.087 (0.019-0.12)	<0.001	0.00	0.006 (0.001-0.02)**	<0.01
tHcy (µmol/L)	20.2 (19.7-26.5)	26.6 (21.6-31.4)	NS	14.8 (12.2-16.7)*	20.1 (18.2-23.0)**	<0.01
NO (µmol/L)	63.2 (59.7-106.2)	28.5 (14.8-46.8)	<0.001	62.4 (49.4-99.1)	36.2 (21.7-49.2)	<0.01
ET-1 (pg/mL)	2.6 (2.2-4.0)	7.0 (4.1-8.8)	<0.001	2.2 (2.0-3.5)	5.7 (4.0-8.0)	<0.001

*Significant difference between without LVH at baseline and after 18 months on PD.
** Significant difference between with LVH at baseline and after 18 months on PD.

LV mass index statistically negatively correlated with serum concentrations of nitric oxide before PD treatment (r = -0.653), and after 18 months on PD (r = -0.759) (p < 0.001) (Figure 3).

A statistically significant positive correlation between left ventricular mass index and serum concentrations of endothelin 1 before PD treatment (r = 0.641) and after 18 months on PD was observed (r = 0.74) (p < 0.001) (Figure 4).

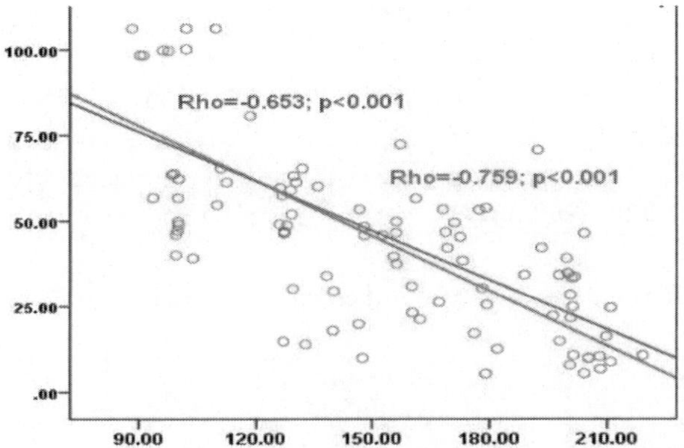

O LVMi and NO at baseline; O LVMi and NO after 18 months PD; / LVMi and NO at baseline; / LVMi and NO after 18 months PD

O LVMi and NO at baseline; O LVMi and NO after 18 months PD;/LVMi and NO at baseline;/LVMi and NO after 18 months PD.

Figure 3. Correlation between LVMi and NO during monitoring period.

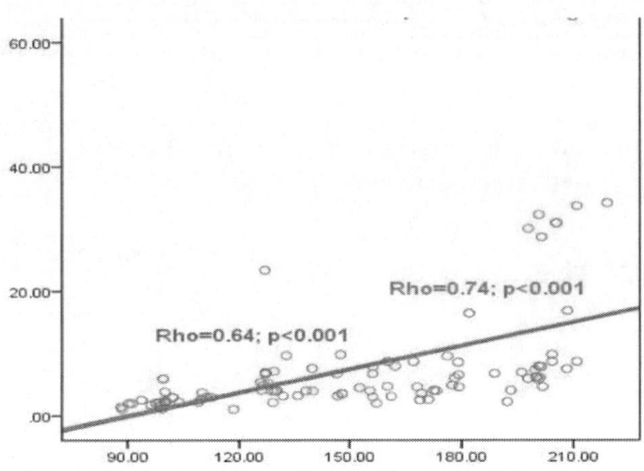

O LVMi and ET-1 at baseline; O LVMi and ET-1 after 18 months PD, / LVMi and ET-1 at baseline; / LVMi and ET-1 after 18 months PD

Figure 4. Correlation between LVMi and ET-1 during monitoring period.

For the purpose of examining independent predictors of stated parameters, we included the following dependent variables in the regression analysis model: blood pressure, DM type 2, body mass index, smoking, sex, age, cholesterol, triglycerides, uremia related parameters (albumin, beta 2-microglobulin, CaxP, CRP, fibrinogen, Hgb, Hct), parameters connected with peritoneal dialysis adequacy (urea, creatinin, diuresis, RRF) and cardiovascular biomarkers(BNP, troponin, ET-1, NO and Hcy).

Independent positive LV mass predictors after 18 months were: cholesterol, apolipoprotein B and diastolic blood pressure, while HDL and NO were independent negative LV mass index predictors. The stated model could be used to explain 70% of result variations ($R^2 = 0.691$) (Table 11).

Table 11. Predictors of LV mass index changes in PD patients

Model	Non standardized coefficients		Standardized coefficients	t	p
	B	Standard error	Beta		
	87.324	38.990		2.240	0.032
Cholesterol	209.166	36.079	0.595	5.797	<0.001
HDL	-110.151	51.287	-0.312	-2.148	0.039
Apo B	27.138	12.863	0.304	2.110	0.042
DBP	207.309	64.137	0.378	3.232	0.003
NO	-58.256	13.770	-0.434	-4.231	<0.001
Dependent variable: Left ventricular mass index					

Note: HDL, high-density lipoprotein; Apo B, apolipoprotein B; DBP, diastolic blood pressure; NO, nitric oxide.

Table 12. Predictors of LV hypertrophy after 18 months of peritoneal dialysis

Model	B	Standard error	p	Exp(B)	95% Confidence Interval	
					Min.	*Max.*
NO	-0.132	0.050	0.009	0.877	0.795	0.967
RRF	-0.002	0.001	0.043	0.244	0.217	0.612
Proteinuria	-0.102	1.001	0.024	14.32	1.641	27.27
CRP	0.453	0.171	0.008	1.572	1.124	2.200
Troponin	95.021	47.860	0.005	1849.0	3.378	1037
LDL	3.604	1.011	0.000	36.734	5.066	266.359
Dependent variable: Left ventricular hypertrophy after 18 months on PD						

Note: NO, nitric oxide; RRF, residual renal function; CRP, C-reactive protein; LDL, low-density lipoprotein.

In a logistical regression analysis model, by examining LVH presence predictors after 18 months of PD treatment, it was determined that CRP, troponin and LDL are independent positive predictors of LV hypertrophy after 18 months of PD treatment, while NO and RRF and proteinuria are independent negative LVH predictors (Table 12.) The model was statistically significant (Chi square = 34.2; $p < 0.001$), and could explain between 50% (R2, Cox and Snell) and 67% (R2 Nagelkerkea) of result variations, and accurately classify 86% of cases.

Carotid Artery and Peritoneal Dialysis

After 18 months of peritoneal dialysis treatment, statistically significant lesser median levels of intimal-medial thickening index of the common carotid arteries were observed (IMT CCA) ($p < 0.001$). Also, medial values of end-diastolic flow velocity (EDV) and peak systolic velocity (PSV) on the CCA are statistically significantly lower after 18 months of PD treatment in relation to basal values ($p < 0.001$) (Table 13).

Table 13. Ultrasound parameters of CCA during monitoring period

	Baseline	18months on PD	p
IMT (mm)	0.73 (0.6-0.9)	0.70 (0.5-0.8)	<0.05
CCA diameter (mm)	5.8 (5.2-6.4)	5.00 (4.9-5.4)	<0.001
Plaque score	4.15 (4.2-5.4)	3.95 (2.9-5.1)	<0.05
EDV (cm/s)	45.0 (35.0-65.0)	38.0 (30.0-50.0)	<0.001
PSV (cm/s)	130.0 (110.0-158.0)	120.0 (98.0-130.0)	<0.001

Note: IMT, intima-media thickness; CCA, common carotid artery; EDV, end-diastolic velocity; PSV, peak systolic velocity.

A statistically significant increase in patient numbers with no verified atherosclerotic plaques on common carotid arteries was observed at the end of monitoring in relation to baseline (26% vs. 44%) (Figure 5).

On the basis of the division of atherosclerotic changes in the CCA by severity in four groups, there was statistically significant lesser number of patients with severe CCA atherosclerosis after 18 months of CAPD treatment. At the beginning of the study 44% of patients suffered from severe atherosclerosis (AS3) while after 18 months of PD treatment it was discovered that only 26% of subjects had severe atherosclerotic changes on the CCA ($p < 0.016$) (Table 14.)

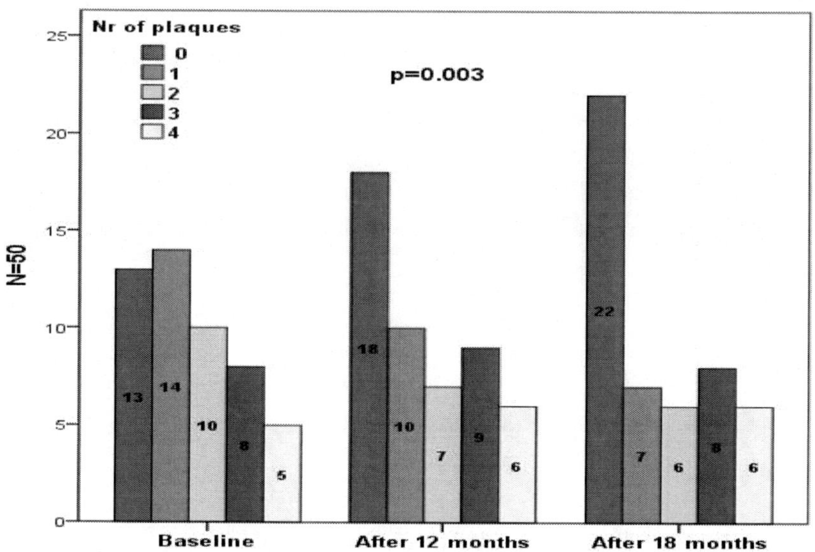

Figure 5. The presentation of atherosclerotic plaques on the CCA during monitoring period.

Table 14. Different PD patient subgroups according to atherosclerotic stage on CCA

	Baseline (n = 50)	12 months PD (n = 50)	18 months PD (n = 50)	p
AS0	16 (32.0%)	16 (32.0%)	19 (38.0%)	0.016
AS1	5 (10%)	7 (14.0%)	8 (16.0%)	
AS2	7 (14.0%)	7 (14.0%)	10 (20.0%)	
AS3	22 (44.0%)	20 (40.0%)	13 (26.0%)	

Statistically significant PCR values varied among groups with different CCA atherosclerosis, both before PD treatment started, and after 18 months on PD treatment (Table 15). There is a significant difference among groups with varying degrees of CCA atherosclerosis in relation to peritoneal dialysis adequacy, and peritoneum transport characteristics. The loss of protein by dialysis effluent has its highest values in the AS3 group (Table 15).

Table 15. The parameters of peritoneal dialysis in different PD patient subgroups according to atherosclerotic stage

		Baseline				18 months PD			
		AS0 (n=16)	AS1/AS2 (n=12)	AS3 (n=22)	p	AS0 (n=19)	AS1/AS2 (n=18)	AS3 (n=13)	p
PCR g/kg/24h		1.0 ±0.1	0.97 ±0.1	0.95 ±0.1	<0.01†	1.14 ±0.1*	1.11 0.1*	1.05 ±0.1*	<0.01†
Protein loss (PD effluent)(g)		2.1 ±1,4	4,2± 0.91	6.9 ±3.1	<0.01†	2.3 ±1.0	4.0 ±1,22	7.0 ±3.7	<0.05 **†┤
Kt/V urea	<1.7	1 (6.3%)	2 (16.6%)	6 (27.3%)	<0.01†	0	1 (5.55%)	5 (38.5%)	<0.01†
	1.7-2.0	6 (37.5%)	8 (66.6%)	14 (18.2%)	<0.01†	10 (52.6%)*	10 (55.5%)*	8 61.5%*	<0.01†
	>2.0	9 (56.3%)	2 (16.6%)	2 (9.1%)	<0.01 **†	9 (47,4%)	0	0	<0.01 **†
Low-average transporters(T) n(%)		12 (75%)	7 (58.3%)	11 (50%)	NS	14 (73.7%)	12 (66.6%)*	3 (23.1%)*	<0.01†
High-average T n(%)		4 (25%)	2 (16.6%)	5 (22.7%)	<0.01 **†	5 (26.3%)	2 (11.1%)	5 (38.5%)	<0.01 **†┤
High T n (%)		0	3 (25%)	8 (36.4%)	<0.01 **†	0	4 (22.2%)	5* (38.5%)	<0.01†

Note: PCR, protein catabolic rate;

* - Significant difference between groups with the same degree of atherosclerosis after 18 months of treatment of PD compared to baseline; **- Significant difference between groups AS1/AS2 and AS0; †- Significant difference between groups AS3 and AS0; ┤- Significant difference between groups AS3 and AS1/AS2; NS-non significant.

Residual renal function (RRF) significantly varied among groups with varying levels of CCA atherosclerosis, both basally ($p < 0.001$) m and after 12 ($p < 0.01$), or 18 months ($p < 0.01$) of peritoneal dialysis treatment. In patients with no CCA atherosclerotic changes (AS0), significantly larger amounts of residual renal function were discovered after 18 months of PD treatment in relation to pre-treatment values ($p < 0.01$) (Figure 6).

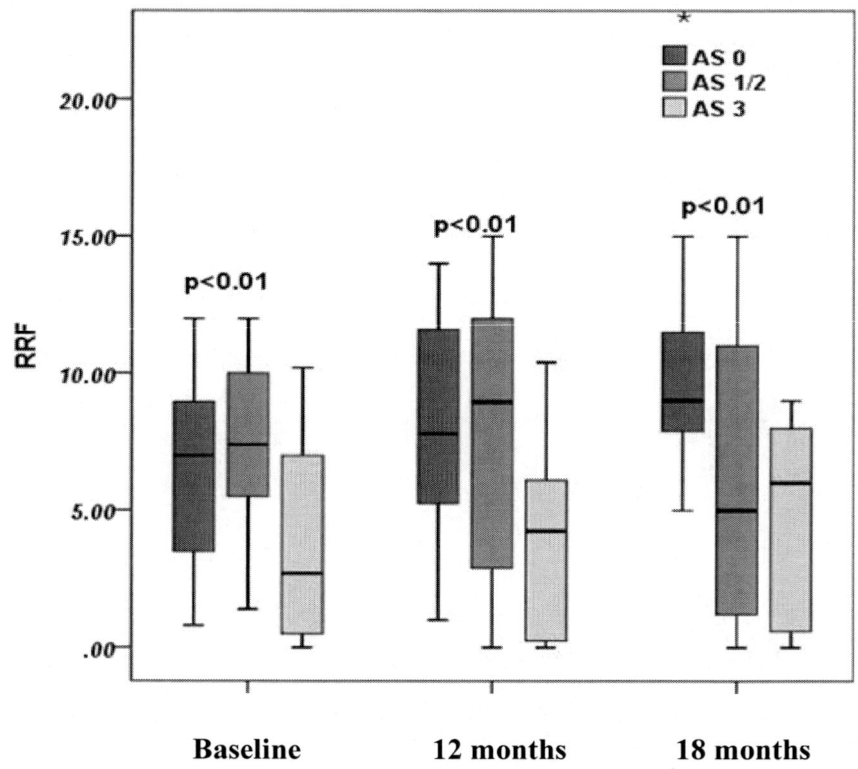

Figure 6. RRF in patients before and after 12 and 18 months of peritoneal dialysis in relation to the stage of atherosclerotic changes in the carotid arteries.

By examining CCA diameter predictors after 18 months of PD treatment in a logistical regression analysis model, it was determined that albumin and Hgb are independent negative, while LDL and age are positive CCA diameter predictors during dialysis treatment. The model was statistically significant (Chi square = 47.9; $p < 0.001$) and could explain the 62% (R2. Cox and Snell) and 82% (R2 Nagaelkerkea) result variations and accurately classify 92% of cases (Table 16).

Table 16. Multiple regression analysis showing factors independently associated with changes of CCA diameter

Model	B	Standard error	p	Exp(B)	95% Confidence Interval	
					Min.	Max.
Albumin	-1.11	0.459	0.015	0.329	0.134	0.809
Hemoglobin	-0.15	0.074	0.037	0.857	0.741	0.991
Low-density lipoprotein	1.402	0.652	0.032	4.063	1.131	.591
Age	0.171	0.078	0.029	1.186	1.018	1.383
Dependent variable: CCA diameter						

Table 17. Multiple regression model of risk factors and their relation to indicators of carotid atherosclerosis in observed ESRD and PD patients

Model	Not standardized coefficients		Standardized coefficients	t	p
	B	Standard error	Beta		
tHCy	0.492	0.079	0.564	6.210	<0.001
CRP	0.142	0.031	0.423	4.615	<0.001
HDL	-0.462	0.111	-0.379	-4.154	<0.001
LDL	0.409	0.133	0.387	3.080	0.004
Lipoprotein (a)	1.604	0.011	0.489	5.066	0.048
CaxP	0.084	0.021	0.349	4.034	<0.001
Endotelin-1	0.134	0.043	0.401	3.115	0.004
Proteinuria	0.402	0.131	0.402	2.097	0.022
Dependent variable: Intima-media thickness of CCA					

Note: tHcy, total homocysteine; CRP, C-reactive protein; HDL, high-density lipoprotein; LDL, low-density lipoprotein;

In a regression analysis model, it was determined that HDL is an independent negative, and that tHCy, CRP, CaxP, ET-1 and LDL are independent positive predictors of IMT CCA, after PD treatment was monitored over a period of 18 months. The suggested model could explain 90% of result variations ($R^2 = 0.90$) (Table 17).

The Relation of Left Ventricular Alterations and Ultrasound Changes of Carotid Arteries in PD Patients

In severe atherosclerosis (AS3) patients, statistically significantly reduced systolic ($p < 0.01$) and diastolic LV function ($p < 0.01$) was observed in relation to the patient group with mild/moderate CCA atherosclerosis (AS1/AS2), as well as in relation to the patient group with no atherosclerosis (AS0) both basally, and after 18 months of PD treatment (Table 18.). A significant progression of LV hypertrophy was observed as well, synchronized with the severity of atherosclerotic carotid artery changes ($p < 0.01$) (Table 18).

5. DISCUSSION

The risk of cardiovascular mortality in dialysis patients is almost 9 times greater than the risk in the general population. Cardiovascular disease is often present in ESRD patients at the inclusion into renal replacement therapy, but can also be developed during chronic dialysis treatment [90]. Dialysis patients suffer 40% mortality because of cardiovascular disease (40% in USA, 36% in Europe) [70]. A study conducted in 2009 on European ESRD patients showed that in dialysis patients the risk of cardiovascular or non-cardiovascular mortality is equally increased in the first three years of dialysis treatment compared to the same diseases in the general population [91], which points to the importance of assessment, as well as precise action on the modification of modifiable CV disease risk factors.

Cardiovascular diseases, be they: congestive failure, myocardial infarction or cardiac arrhythmias, are most often the consequence of LVH or left ventricular dilatation, and ischemic heart disease. Verifying LV disorders by Doppler echocardiography is an important step in the characterization of patients towards CV risk, the assessment of the presence of primary cardiac disease, the function of predisposing factors and the prognostic assessment of their influences, as well as monitoring the effectiveness of therapeutic interventions. A Canadian study showed that out of 432 patients in ESRD before the start of dialysis treatment, only 16% of patients had a normal echocardiogram [92].In a multicentric, prospective study by Nardi and associates in 2007, LVH was verified in 74% of patients immediately before the start of renal replacement therapy.

Table 18. The relationship between echocardiographic parameters in PD patients according to the stage of atherosclerotic changes in the carotid arteries

	Baseline				After 18 months on PD			
	AS0 (n=16)	AS1/AS2 (n=12)	AS3 (n=22)	p	AS0 (n=19)	AS1/AS2 (n=18)	AS3 (n=13)	p
EF (%)	56.59 ±7	52.10 ±8.4	44.32 ±7.9	p < 0.01†**	62.37 ±8.2	57.39 ±9.7	48.38 ±6.9	p < 0.01 †**
E/A	1.04 ±.1	0.98 ±0.1	0.89 ±0.1	p < 0.01**	1.14 ±0.1	1.10 ±0.1	1.02 ±.0	p < 0.01 †**
LVEDD (mm)	51.09 ±2.9	50.72 ±1.4	55.36 ±3.5	p < 0.01†**	46.38 ±8.8	49.71 ±2.5	54.19 ±3.2	p < 0.01 †
LVMi (g/m^2)	149.52 ±34.9	152.74 ±40.0	176.58 ±36.0	p < 0.01**	119.5 ±29.6	137.93 ±31.1	173.75 ±35. 3	p < 0.01 *†**
LVM (gr)	261.30 ±36.4	275.22 ±28.2	297.80 ±48.7	p < 0.01**	221.31 ±26.1	248.05 ±38.8	270.95 ±44.8	p < 0.01 *,**
LVV (mL)	76.10 ±20.1	83.03 ±16.6	104.28 ±24.0	p < 0.01†**	72.83 ±17.0	80.16 ±17.1	105.0 ±19.1	p < 0.01 †**
LAD (mm)	40.10 ±4.1	41.17 ±3.4	46.90 ±5.8	p < 0.01†**	37.98 ±8.5	40.45 ±3.7	44.1 ±5.3	p < 0.01 *†**
FS (%)	32.40 ±3.6	30.27 ±3.8	25.46 ±4.7	p < 0.01†**	33.49 ±3.2	30.61 ±4.0	27.21 ±2.6	p < 0.01*†**

Note: EF, ejection fraction; LVEDD, left ventricular end. diastolic diameter; LVMI- LV mass index; LVM, LV mass; LVV, LV volume; LAD, left atrium diameter; FS, fractional shortening.

* - Significant difference between groups AS1/AS2 and AS0; **- Significant difference between groups AS3 and AS0;

†- Significant difference between groups AS3 and AS1/AS2.

By analyzing and modifying the left ventricular, we determined the presence of LVH in 39/50 (78%) of patients before their inclusion in the dialysis treatment program. Such results correlate with the above stated research results. A high percentage of LVH patients suggests that predisposing LVH factors are present, and that they function even in the IV stage of chronic kidney disease.

After 18 months of PD treatment, through echocardiographic analysis, we discovered LVH in 60% of subjects, while 40% subjects had a normal cardiac ultrasound. 18% more patients had normal LV structure after 18 months on PD. Such a result could be explained by significant volume unburdening, anemia correction, good hypertension control, but also the positive effects of adequate peritoneal dialysis on modifying the function of a series of hemodynamic and non-hemodynamic cardiovascular risk factors in this population.

Carotid ultrasonography is a basal technique of high sensitivity for the examination of the vascular system. The estimation of carotid artery changes by this technique is important not only for the evaluation of its structural changes, but also for the evaluation of atherosclerosis of the complete vascular system. Intima-media thickness, particularly on CCA, is a strong predictor of cardiovascular changes in the general population. Because of this it is considered today to be an important surrogate marker of atherosclerosis and outcome measure of tracking in interventionist studies, directed at the modification of cardiovascular risk factors.

Studies based on ultrasonography of CCA in ESRD patients have determined the existence of significant arterial damage [93]. Blacher and associates discovered that internal CCA diameter in renal failure is a marker of arterial rigidity, and an independent predictor of total mortality [94]. Research by Benedetto and associates showed that the primary negative effect on the complete cardiovascular system, observed through CCA changes, are not only changes in wall thickness, the presence of atherosclerotic plaques or changes in CCA diameter, but also the rigidity of the arterial tree wall, which is a consequence of structural changes on these blood vessels [94]. By the study conducted, we have determined that the average CCA wall thickening, measured by IMT, before the start of PD treatment, was 0.73 mm, with a range of values between 0.6 to 0.9 mm. The internal CCA diameter was basally 5.8 mm (range 5.2-6.4 mm). In research conducted by Stompor and associates, in patients who were already included in the PD treatment program, average IMT was 0.75 ± 0.17 mm (49). While the results of the Italian authors [95] prove that the average CCA diameter in ESRD patients who were already included in a program of dialysis treatment (HD, PD) was 6.86 ± 0.92 mm, which is more than in our subjects. The same authors did not find atherosclerotic plaques in 26 subjects (25%), while there were 50% with 1-4 atherosclerotic plaques, and 25% of subjects with 4 or more. In our research, which differed in subject number, but also in the fact that basal parameters were measured immediately before inclusion into the PD treatment program, we verified 26% of patients had no plaques, 64% with 1-4 plaques, while 10% of monitored patients had 4 or more atherosclerotic plaques. We basally calculated the CCA plaque score, which was 4.15 (range 4.2-5.4).

Functional CCA status was estimated based on the value of peak systolic velocity (PSV), which averaged over the top referential boundary, that is 130cm/s (range 110 -158 cm/s), while end diastolic velocity (EDV) averaged on the lower boundary of normal values, which is 45 cm/s. At the beginning of peritoneal dialysis treatment, 32% of patients had no ultrasound signs of CCA atherosclerosis, 24% had mild/moderate atherosclerosis (AS1/AS2), while 44% of patients were in the severe atherosclerosis (AS3) group. These results contribute to the assumption that the atherosclerotic process in ESRD patients is extremely present and advanced even before renal replacement therapy.

After 18 months of monitoring, the average IMT CCA was 0.70 mm with a significant reduction of CCA diameter (5.0 mm). The calculated CCA plaque score was somewhat reduced and at the end of observation was 3.95. Hemodynamic parameters of ultrasound of the CCA show a statistically significant reduction of systolic and diastolic flow, which leads to the conclusion that hemodynamic parameters of CCA in patients treated by PD were significantly better, and consequently arterial wall rigidity is lessened. The ration of patients without verified atherosclerotic CCA plaques after 18 months is significantly greater in relation to the basal result (26% vs. 44%).

Caliskan and associates [96] in their research determined that the average IMT CCA is 1.05 mm after including ESRD patients in PD treatment programs, while Stompor and associates [23], after a yearly observation of PD treated patients, determined that the IMT value (0.66 vs. 0.75 mm) was significantly reduced, along with a smaller number of subjects with atherosclerotic CCA plaques (40.4 vs. 59.6%), which agrees with the results achieved in this research.

The changes in the vascular system in uremic patients are attributed to a synergetic function of several factors, which modify structural and functional characteristics of the vascular system [8]. Meeus and associates pointed to a high occurrence of atherosclerosis in chronic kidney disease patients, and assumed that the process of atherosclerosis in ESRD is accelerated [14].

Atherosclerosis and arterial remodeling are, first and foremost, connected to aging (arteriosclerosis) and hemodynamic changes. Arterial remodeling was observed in patients at the very start of CKD, after the inclusion into renal replacement therapy programs, and is comparable to patients treated by both forms of dialysis. This points to the conclusion that non-hemodynamic factors can play an important role in the pathophysiology of vascular complication origin [97].

In Benedetto and associates survey [98] on patients treated by HD or PD, the second measurement of CCA diameter after 12 months of treatment showed a statistically nonsignificant smaller CCA diameter in relation to baseline (6.88 vs. 6.86 mm). Mutluay and associates in their study, conducted over 24 months, established that IMT is an independent predictor of cardiovascular mortality, regardless of dialysis form, with a high prevalence of advanced atherosclerotic process, traced through structural changes on CCA, but also with the positive effect of dialysis treatment alone, which is reflected on partial CCA changes regression [99].

In the USA, more than half of ESRD patients have some form of cardiovascular disease (e.g., cardiac arrest, coronary disease, peripheral vessel disease), present prior to the start of renal replacement therapy, while newly diagnosed cardiovascular diseases are being developed at the rate of 10% a year [100]. According to that, it would be useful to ascertain what is the contribution of general risk factors for the development of cardiovascular disease, risk factors relevant to ESRD, and risk factors specifically relevant to chronic PD. It was also important to estimate whether treating PD patients changes modifiable CV risk factors positively, or negatively.

Cardiovascular diseases are attributed to half of the general mortality of dialysis patients, and the ratio increases with the increase of life expectancy [101]. Age is an irreversible traditional risk factor for the development of cardiovascular disease in the general population, as well as in uremic patients. In our research, the average age of subjects is 60.5 (26-76), with a balanced sex representation. Diabetic nephropathy was the cause of ESRD in 48% of patients.

According to epidemiological studies data, arterial hypertension is represented in around 50% of peritoneal dialysis patients, and up to 80% in hemodialysis patients. The European Society of Hypertension (ESH/ASC) in their 2013 guidelines, included hypertension among the main CV risk factors with chronic kidney disease [102]. Arterial hypertension has an influence on the development of LVH, congestive heart failure and atherosclerosis. Heerspink and associates meta-analysis gave the basis for the assumption that proper treatment of PD patients with antihypertensives, primarily ACE inhibitors and angiotensin II receptor blockers, directly influences better survival rates [24]. Guidelines by Kidney Disease Outcome Quality Initiative (K/DOQI) recommend maintaining blood pressure in dialysis patients to values less than 140/90mm Hg [103].

During our research, a significant drop in SBP in PD patients occurred, which at the start of the study, according to actual classifications, was in the range of first-degree hypertension (147.4 vs. 129.4 mmHG, $p < 0.001$). DBP was also significantly reduced, in relation to basal values (85.2 vs. 78.4 mmHg, $p < .0.001$). Numerous studies have pointed out the connection between high blood pressure and LVH [104]. The conducted research has confirmed significant differences in median values of SBP, DBP and mean BP between groups with and without LVH, at the start of the treatment, as well as after 18 months of peritoneal dialysis treatment. We have also determined that high DBP presents a strong independent left ventricular mass index predictor. Tonbul and associates found similar results in their research, determining that there are significant differences in groups with and without LVH according to blood pressure values [105]. Earlier research had given the basis for the conclusion that antihypertensive therapy leads to LVH regression, and so reduces the risk connected to increased left ventricular mass [90]. Volume unburdening and adequate depuration of PD patients plays a major role in the correction of arterial hypertension, which, according to Laplace's norm, reduces burden and LV tension, and creates the conditions for the regression of its remodeling process.

Dyslipidemia is a traditional modifiable cardiovascular disease risk factor in the general population [106, 107]. We have determined that dyslipidemia in our PD patients was permanently present, primarily at the expense of increased total cholesterol and triglyceride values. Changes in the metabolism of monitored lipoprotein fractions were observed (drop of Lp (a) levels, significantly reduced apoB levels, and the increase of apoA 1 levels). Similar results were published by other authors [106, 108]. It is necessary to point out that in patients treated by PD, a series of other factors, specific to this type of dialysis, can affect serum lipid levels, particularly secondary hyperparathyroidism, insulin resistance, peritoneal glucose absorption, and finally renal disease etiology itself. A group of subject with LVH at the start of the study had significantly greater total cholesterol and triglyceride levels in serum, in relation to the subject group with no LVH. This ratio was sustained up to the end of the study. Longenecker and associates, in the CHOICE study, determined that serum lipid levels, in interaction with other, non-tradition

CVD risk factors, are significantly connected to LVH [107]. On the other hand PD itself is connected to a relatively aterogenic lipid profile in relation to the general populations, but also hemodialysis patients. It is assumed that the reason for this is stimulation of liver synthesis of lipoproteins following glucose absorption from the dialysis solution, increased insulin levels, as well as selective loss of protein via dialysis effluent, which is quantitatively analogous to nephrotic syndrome. In our study, we have discovered that total cholesterol and apolipoprotein B are independent positive predictors of left ventricular mass index in PD patients. It is known that apoB is connected to coronary heart disease in the general population, while in dialysis patients it is still subject to debate, and various controversies. Its role in PD patients as CVD factor has so far not been examined, and so the result of a statistically significant independent combination of average concentration of apo B in serum and LV mass index can provide a foundation for further studies into its role in LV remodeling.

In our study, serum lipid levels are continuously increased in all patient groups classified according to the severity of the atherosclerotic process (AS0, AS1, AS2, AS3). An independent positive combination of LDL and a negative combination of HDL with IMT CCA after 18 months of PD treatment, supports the claim of Cengis and associates [108] that changes on CCA are tied to a disturbed lipid profile, primarily through the reduction of HDL levels, as well as the increase of LDL levels, which contributes to the atherosclerotic process, which is clearly witnessed in CCA structural changes by measured IMT. With the conducted research, we have confirmed that HDL presents a significant independent factor, which influences LVH regression, and CCA IMT in peritoneal dialysis patients. On the other hand, we confirmed that LDL has a significant effect as a predictor to the development of LVH and an increase of carotid arterial wall rigidity. These results contribute to the current position, that in dialysis patients, lipid disruption should be treated aggressively, to reduce the risk of CV diseases and sustain LDL levels at less than 3 mmol/L [109, 110].

Anemia is one of the primary markings of the ESRD, and is a risk factor of cardiovascular diseases connected to uremic mileu. Generally it is the consequence of reduced erythropoietin hormone secretion in the kidneys, as the most significant erythropoietin regulator. Anemia leads to reduced oxygen content per the unit of blood volume and condition of relative tissue hypoxia. Reduced oxygen intake causes local vasodilation, which significantly increases preload and minute volume, as a compensatory mechanism of reduced oxygen transport capacity. This increase of minute volume with the aim of satisfying metabolic needs reflects on LV structure [111]. The results of a large prospective multi-centric study by Canadian authors, which encompassed a group of 432 ESRD patients with several unwanted outcomes, showed cardiomyopathy, cardiac dysfunction and death, independently of other risk factors. The same authors determined that the drop in hemoglobin levels of 1g/L is connected to significant risk increase of the development of LV dilation, de novo, and recurring cardiac insufficiency [112]. Our study of hemoglobin values at the end of the observation period showedresults significantly greater in relation to starting results (118.6 vs. 101.9 g/L, p < 0,001). This can primarily be explained by substitutive erythropoietin treatment, with which all subjects were treated (average 6000 IU s.c. per week), with consequential increase of erythrocyte mass. Appropriate PD treatment contributed to the modification of the response to this hormone therapy. In relation to LVH presence in basal results, we have determined that there is no statistically significant difference in hemoglobin levels between LVH and non LVH subject groups, but also that at the end of observation, there was a statistically significant difference in hemoglobin levels in groups with different LV hypertrophy types (concentric and eccentric LVH).

The connection of malnutrition, inflammation, and atherosclerosis forms a special syndrome, the so called MIA syndrome, which is very common in PD patients. Chronic inflammation apparently contributes to accelerated atherosclerosis and the development of malnutrition syndrome. There are two types of MIA syndrome: MIA type 1 marked by insufficient protein-energy intake, and is rarely connected to CVD development. Type 2 MIA syndrome develops with chronic inflammation and points to a significant correlation between increased atherosclerosis levels and CVD. PD patients generally have reduced levels of serum albumin and an increase of C reactive protein value [113]. In our study, at the start of evaluation and before inclusion into PD treatment program, albumin levels in serum were significantly lower in relation to albumin levels at the end of study (p < 001). The loss of protein through urine in patients with preserved residual renal function after 18 months of observation are smaller in relation to basal median values, and the difference is at the very edge of statistical significance (p = 0.05). In PD patients, the loss of protein through dialysis effluent after the first 6 months and after 18 months of PD treatment averaged 6.4 g/L/24 hours, while protein degradation speed averaged 0.9-1.0 g/kg/24h. This data points to a milder severity of patient malnutrition in our subjects, as well as on the samples of this malnutrition. By applying the logistical regression analysis model, we have determined that after 18 months of observation, proteinuria is a negative predictor of LVH in PD patients. It was also discovered that low levels of albumin in serum are an independent negative predictor of common carotid artery diameter, which is the rigidity of the arterial wall, and proteinuria is a determinant of structural changes on the CCA wall, particularly in severe atherosclerosis patients. In a study conducted by Szeto and associates on PD patients over 3 years, it was discovered that albumin levels in serum, and the loss of protein by dialysate are significant independent predictors of CV complications in PD patients [114].

By researching endothelial dysfunction in dialysis patients, which leads to structural changes of the vascular tree and consequential clinical readings on CV system, Stenvinkel and associates have discovered that endothelial dysfunction is connected to reduced bioavailability of NO, and increased levels of his endogen inhibitor, which is increased concentration of ADMA in serum, which further leads to increased vascular rigidity and CV mortality risk [115]. Endothelial dysfunction in uremia patients is also connected to higher levels of fibrinogen in plasma, CRP, endothelin and other factors. In a study by Wang and associates [116] it was determined that CRP levels can be a predictor of cardiac changes in dialysis patients. In this research, there is an inverse relation between inflammation and RRF in PD patients and anuric PD patients had a greater level of serum CRP in relation to patients with preserved RRF.

In our research we have determined that CRP and fibrinogen values, as factors of CV risk after 18 months of PD treatment, were statistically significantly lower in patients with normal LV and in the subject group with no carotid artery atherosclerotic changes in relation to other observed groups. CRP values in serum are an independent significant predictor of LVH ($p = 0.008$). IMT CCA ($p < 0.001$). These results give the foundation for the conclusion that inflammatory factors are certainly involved in changes to LV structure, but also with the development of atherosclerotic process on common carotid arteries. However there is still no proposed, or generally accepted manner of treatment for chronic PD patient inflammation.

Increased levels of serum phosphate and CaxP product are known risk factors of CV morbidity and mortality, both in HD and PD patients [117] who increase the risk of the creation of calcifications in blood vessels on valves and in tissues. Even though hyperphosphatemia is considered a relatively rare complication in PD patients, the results of several studies point to the fact that it is very diverse in PD population. A NECOSAD study [117] and survey from Wang and associates [116] has shown that around 40% of chronic PD patients have serum levels of phosphate above the targeted value of 1.78 mmol/L, which is recommended by KDOQI. Our research has shown that phosphate and CaxP product values are statistically significantly greater in LVH patients in relation to subjects with normal LV morphology. Such results were achieved both basally and after 18 months of dialysis treatment. Achieved results were in accordance with a large prospective NECOSAD study [51], where an independent combination of increased phosphate concentration in serum and CaxP product was found, with cardiovascular morbidity, specifically with vascular calcifications and LVH, but not with iPTH concentration.

Residual renal function is very important for PD patients, because it contributes to total daily clearance by 20% and more, as well as to the control of volume status [118]. Basal results of our research show that there was no statistically significant difference between patients with verified LVH and patients with normal LV in size calculated residual renal function, and not in total daily diuresis volume either. However after 18 months of PD treatment LVH patients had significantly worse residual renal function in relation to subjects with normal LV (5.1. vs. 9.8 ml/min). The same relation was noted in daily urine collection. In LVH patients daily diuresis was 376.3 ml/24h, while in patients with no LVH it was 897.5 ml/24h. Using the logistical regression analysis model, examining LVH predictors after 18 months of peritoneal dialysis treatment, residual renal function has shown itself to be a significant independent LVH predictor. This result strongly supports the hypothesis of the negative effects of drop of loss of residual renal function of CV morbidity, which agrees with the results of several large randomized studies conducted on PD patients [76-78]. In our study, the total volume of daily diuresis is shown as an independent determinant of diastolic LV dysfunction in PD patients, which is according to studies by Konings and Wang [119].

Morphological-functional LV changes can be observed by determining the level of circulatory BNP. It has been determined that BNP levels in plasma are significantly greater in patients treated by HD and PD, particularly in HD patients in relation to patients with CKD, as well as LVH in dialysis patients [120, 121]. That kind of result points to a synergistic action of the loss of renal function, and an increase of circulating BNP levels in induction and creation of LVH. An ADEMEX study showed that BNP levels are independent markers of survival in the PD population [120]. In our research, we have determined that average BNP values in ESRD patients were significantly more in relation to values after 18 months of peritoneal dialysis treatment (p < 0.001). Echocardiographic analysis showed that LVH patients have significantly higher values of BNP than subjects with no LVH, particularly in the eccentric LVH group. A positive correlation of BNP with followed LV morphology parameters was observed, but also parameters of systolic and diastolic LV function both at the beginning and after 18 months of PD treatment.

By observing the connection of homocysteine concentrations in serum and carotid artery atherosclerosis we have determined that statistically significantly larger values of homocysteine in patients with ultrasound determined severe atherosclerosis in relation to patients with no/mild/moderate CCA atherosclerosis. By the regression analysis, we determined that homocysteine is an independent predictor of structural changes in the CCA wall, which is IMT CCA ($p < 0.001$). The Yilmaz and associates survey confirmed a positive correlation of homocysteine with IMT CCA. The role of homocysteine as an independent risk factor for CCA atherosclerotic changes in patients on peritoneal dialysis was not determined in that study.

Endothelial function is damaged in both patients on hemodialysis and peritoneal dialysis, most likely because of the reduced bioavailability of nitric oxide. The resulting research pointed out that NO production in peritoneal dialysis patients is low [65]. However, their results of our longitudinal study point out that average NO value was significantly greater after 12, or 18 months of dialysis treatment in relation to basal results ($p < 0.001$). Subjects with normal echocardiographic LV results have significantly greater NO values at the start, but after 18 months of PD treatment as well. Our results are in line with results from Foud and associates, which were that levels of serum NO negatively correlate with LVMI in dialysis patients (208). It was discovered by regressive analysis that NO is a statistically significant independent negative LV mass index predictor ($p < 0.001$) of LVH ($p = 0.009$), which aids the strong connection of NO levels with LV morphological changes in PD patients, giving them the function of an "antihyperthrophic" molecule.

In response to mechanical and chemical stimulations, endothelial cells react by creating a series of biologically active compounds, including endothelial relaxation factor, nitric oxide, but also a vasoconstrictive factor – endothelin-1. The levels of ET-1 in serum are particularly increased in dialysis patients. However, the mechanisms and meaning of this increase in peritoneal dialysis patients have not been completely cleared, and there are no relevant studies that have dealt with endothelin-1 and cardiovascular changes of this patient population. With the conducted research we have determined that the average value of ET-1 after 18 months of PD treatment was statistically lower in relation to vassal values and values after 12 months of dialysis ($p < 0.01$).

[8]   Ronco, C; Dell'Aquila, R; Rodighiero, MP. Peritoneal dialysis: A clinical update congestive heart failure and PD. *Contrib Nephrol.* 2006, 150, 129-134.

[9]   Larsen, T; Narala, K; McCullough, AP. Type 4 Cardiorenal Syndrome: Myocardial Dysfunction, Fibrosis, and Heart Failure in Patients with Chronic Kidney Disease. *J Clinic Experiment Cardiol.* 2012, 3,186-190.

[10]   Foley, NR; Bryan, M; Curtis, MB; Randell, WE; Parfrey, SP. Left Ventricular Hypertrophy in New Hemodialysis Patients without Symptomatic Cardiac Disease. *Clin J Am Soc Nephrol.* 2010, 5(5), 805-813.

[11]   Cottone, S; Mule, G; Guarneri, M; Palermo, A; Lorito, MC; Riccobene, R. Endothelin-1 and F2-isoprostane relate to and predict renal dysfunction in hypertensive patients. *Nephrol Dial Transplant.* 2009, 24, 497-503.

[12]   Nardi, E; Cottone, S; Mule, G; Palermo, A; Cusimano, P; Cerasola, G. Influence of chronic renal insufficiency on left ventricular diastolic function in hypertensives without left ventricular hypertrophy. *J Nephrol.* 2007, 20, 320-328.

[13]   Nardi, E; Palermo, A; Mule, G; Cusimano, P; Cottone, S; Cerasola, G. Left ventricular hypertrophy and geometry in hypertensive patients with chronic kidney disease. *J Hypertens.* 2009, 27, 633-641.

[14]   Meeus, F; Kourilsky, O; Guerin, AP; Gaudry, C; Marchais, SJ; London, GM. Pathophysiology of cardiovascular disease in hemodialysis patients. *Kidney Int.* 2000, 76, S140-147.

[15]   Meeus, F; Kourilsky, O; Guerin, AP; Gaudry, C; Marchais, SJ; London, GM. Pathophysiology of cardiovascular disease in hemodialysis patients. *Kidney Int.* 2000, 76, S140-147.

[16]   Wang, MC; Tsai, WC; Chen, JY; Cheng, MF; Huang, JJ. Arterial stiffness correlated with cardiac remodelling in patients with chronic kidney disease. *Nephrology (Carlton).* 2007, 12, 591-597.

[17]   Lopez, B; Gonzalez, A; Lsarte, JJ. Is plasma cardiotrophin-1 a marker of hypertensive heart disease? *J Hypertens.* 2005, 23, 625-632.

[18]   Moe, SM; Chen, NX. Mechanisms of Vascular Calcification in Chronic Kidney Disease. *J Am Soc Nephrol.* 2008, 19(2), 213-216.

[19]   London, GM; Marchais, SJ; Guerin, AP; Metivier, F. Arteriosclerosis, vascular calcifications and cardiovascular disease in uremia. *Curr Opin Nephrol Hypertens.* 2005, 14, 525-531.

[20]   London, MG. Vascular disease and atherosclerosis in uremia. Nephrologia. 2005, 25(2), 91-95.

The LVH patient group had significantly greater values of ET-1 in serum, in relation to patients without LVH (p < 0.001). Demuth and associates determined that ET-1 values in hemodialysis patient serum were significantly greater in relation to healthy subjects [121], with a significant positive correlation between HLK and ET-1 in serum, but with no significant connection to functional LV parameters.

By examining the potential role of serum endothelin-1 in vascular remodeling in PD patients, we have determined that ET-1 serum values in basal measurement were statistically significantly greater in patients with severe atherosclerosis, in relation to patients without and patients with mild/moderate atherosclerotic changes. This kind of relation is followed after 18 months of dialysis treatment. Endothelin-1 in serum was positively correlated with structural and hemodynamic parameters of CCA at the start and at the end of the observation period. In logistical regression analysis, we have determined that ET-1 is an independent positive predictor of IMT CCA. The results of this research point to a conclusion that ET-1 concentration in serum presents one of the more important factors, which was tightly tied to the advancement of atherosclerosis in patients on peritoneal dialysis, so that ET-1 could be a biomarker of carotid artery atherosclerosis. ET-1 has an important role in the preservation of blood pressure and the origin of arterial rigidity, which again contributes to oxidative stress, and vascular inflammation, and in the long term to arterial remodeling.

Transport characteristics of peritoneum are the most important optimal PD determinants. The efficiency of peritoneal dialysis is conducted through the PET test (peritoneal equilibration test), although a study by van Biesen determined that PDC (personalized dialysis capacity) gives more information on the markings of the peritoneal membrane, particularly in the presence of an actual inflammation, and quick transportation status. By estimating the adequacy of peritoneal dialysis in the first 6 months of treatment, we determined that around 50% had adequate dialysis (Kt/V urea>2.0) Kt/V in the range of 1.7-2.0 had 42% of patients, while an inadequate dialysis was taken by only 8% of patients through a weekly Kt/V urea. Considering that there were no anuric subjects, this kind of disease distribution could be explained with high malnutrition levels, which is first and foremost reflected in hypoalbuminemia, relatively high diabetic patients in the study, as well as the reduced protein catabolic rate (PCR) at baseline. After 18 months, dialysis treatment was inadequate in only 2% of subjects, 60% of subjects had excellent treatment, and 38% had partially good dialysis adequacy. These results, among others, could be the reason for an individualized, adaptable, and regression of cardiovascular remodelling. Better control of BP and good volume control leads to significant improvements in cardiac function and arterial stiffness. Also, significant presences of cardiovascular modified in ESRD suggests the significance of recognizing and correcting cardiovascular system disorders and risk factors in the early stages of chronic kidney disease. The right choice of targeted pharmacological intervention, with the usage of biocompatible dialysis solutions, the preservation of satisfactory adequacy of dialysis, and transport characteristics of peritoneum, as well as reduced protein loss through dialysis effluent can have a significant effect on cardiovascular remodelling regression in peritoneal dialysis patients, primarily LVH, and atherosclerotic changes on the vascular system.

The results suggest several novel modifiable mechanisms related to the short-term effects of dialysis that are potentially implicated in the development of uremic cardiomyopathy.

REFERENCES

[1]   Bauml, MA; Underwood, DA. Left ventricular hypertrophy: An overlooked cardiovascular risk factor. *Cleve Clin J Med.* 2010, 77(6), 381-387.

[2]   Cerasola, G; Nardi, E; Palermo, A; Mule, G; Cottone, C. Epidemiology and pathophysiology of left ventricular abnormalities in chronic kidney disease: a review. *J Nephrol.* 2011, 24(01), 1-10.

[3]   London, GN. Cardiovascular disease in chronic renal failure:pathophysiologic aspects. *Semin Dial.* 2003, 16, 85-94.

[4]   Schiffrin, EL, Lipman, ML, Mann, JF. Chronic kidney disease:effects on the cardiovascular system. *Circulation.* 2007, 116, 85-97.

[5]   Stewart, GA; Mark, PB; Rooney, E; McDonagh, TA; Dargie, HJ; Staurt, R. Electrocardiographic abnormalities and uremic cardiomyopathy. *Kidney Int.* 2005, 67(1), 217-26.

[6]   Go, AS, Chertow, GM; Fan, D; McCulloch, CE, Hsu, CY. Chronic kidney disease and the risks of death, cardiovascular events, and hospitalization. *N Engl J Med.* 2004, 351(13), 1296-1305.

[7]   Zoccali, C; Mallamaci, F; Benedetto, FA; Tripepi, G; Parlongo, S; Cataliotti, A. Creed Investigators. Cardiac natriuretic peptides are related to left ventricular mass and function and predict mortality in dialysis patients. *J Am Soc Nephrol.* 2001, 12(7), 1508-1515.

flexible manner of dialysis prescription. In PD patients with normal LV there was no inadequate dialysis observed through the Kt/V urea parameter. In a group of LVH subjects, 10.3% of patients had Kt/V < 1.7, while the greatest representation was in the Kt/V 1.7 to 2.0. After 18 months about 95% of patients without LVH had Kt/V > 2.0, while in the LVH group 36.7% of LVH patients had Kt/V > 2.0, and 60% 1.7-2.0.

A significant difference in patient distribution was spotted with or without LVH according to PET test results, which we used to evaluate peritoneum transport characteristics. For the first 6 months of CAPD treatment, 100% of non-LVH patients had low-average peritoneum transport characteristics, while 41% of LVH patients had high-average, or high peritoneum transport characteristics. A similar result was determined after 18 months of CAPD treatment, when 46.7% of LVH patients had high-average or high peritoneum transport characteristics.

Considering the role of volume encumbrance, ultrafiltration deficit, and protein loss through dialysis effluent, the results we have achieved point to the fact that high transporters have a very high prevalence of LVH, conditioned by the function of a series of factors, with no independent influence of the peritoneum transport characteristics themselves. Similar results were published by Huang in 2013, in a two year study of the relation of PD parameters and LV function, determining that patients with no LV dysfunction had significantly better dialysis parameters during the observation period, while patients with reduced LV function had Kt/V less than 2.0 and belonged to the high-average peritoneum transport characteristics group [122].

Inability to achieve total regression of cardiovascular remodeling through dialysis and medication, irrelevant of the achieved partial modification of parts of currently examined traditional and non-traditional risk factors, point to a pathogenic role of unexamined, additional factors. The question of an ideal prognostic biomarker remains unanswered. The effects of new, still hypothetical, CV disease risk factors on the cardiovascular system, such as fetuin A, FGF23, E- selectin osteoprotegerin, hepatocyte growth factor, ICAM1/VCAM1, IL-18, myeloperoxidase, pentraxin 3, TNF, and a series of other factors recognized in experimental studies, remain a subject of further research, with a significant need to examine the total multifactorial effect on the cardiovascular system in peritoneal dialysis patients.

In conclusion, LVH, increased IMT and CCA diameter, impaired diastolic function and normal systolic function are highly present in uremic patients before initiation of renal replacement therapy. PD in the first 18 months of treatment has a positive effect on stopping or even on achieving partial

[21] Jang, JS; Kwon, SK; Kim, HY. Comparison of blood pressure control and left ventricular hypertrophy in patients on continuous ambulatory peritoneal dialysis (CAPD) and automated peritoneal dialysis (APD). *Electrolyte Blood Press.*, 2011, 9, 16-22.

[22] Vanholder, R; Glorieux, G; Lameire, N. for the European Uremic Toxin Work Group (EUTox). Uraemic toxins and cardiovascular disease. *Nephrol Dial Transplant*, 2003, 18, 463-466.

[23] Stompor, T; Krasniak, A; Sulowicz, W; Kieć, DA; Janda, K; Wojcik, K. Changes in common arotid artery intima-media thickness over 1-year in patients on peritoneal dialysis. *Nephrol Dial Transplant.*, 2005, 20 (2), 404-412.

[24] Heerspink, HJ; Ninomiya, T; Zoungas, S; de Zeeuw, D; Grobbee, DE; Jardine, MJ. Effect of lowering blood pressure on cardiovascular events and mortality in patients on dialysis: a systematic review and meta-analysis of randomized controlled trials. *Lancet.*, 2009, 373, 1009–1015.

[25] Tomiyama, C; Higa, A; Dalboni, MA; Cenderogio, M; Draibe, AS; Cuppari, L. The impact of traditional and non-traditional risk factors on coronary calcification in pre-dialysis patients. *Nephrol Dial Transplant.* 2006, 21, 2464-2471.

[26] Weiner, DE; Tighiouart, H; Amin, MG; Griffith, JL; Stark, PC; MacLeod, BD. Chronic kidney disease as a risk factor for cardiovascular disease and all-cause mortality: a pooled analysis of community-based studies. *J Am Soc Nephrol.*, 2004, 15, 1307-1315.

[27] Coen, G; Manni, M; Mantella, D; Pierantozzi, A; Balducci, A; Condo, S. Are PTH serum levels predictive of coronary calcifications in haemodialysis patients? *Nephrol Dial Transplant.*, 2007, 22(11), 3262-3267.

[28] Levey, AS; Coresh, J; Greene, T; Marsh, J; Stevens, AL; Kusek, WJ. Chronic Kidney Disease Epidemiology Collaboration. Expressing the Modification of Diet in Renal Disease Study equation for estimating glomerular filtration rate with standardized serum creatinine values. *Clin Chem.*, 2007, 53, 766-772.

[29] Zoccali, C; Mallamaci, F; Tripepi, G. Novel cardiovascular risk factors in end-stage renal disease. *J Am Soc Nephrol.*, 2004, 15(1), 77-80.

[30] Zoccali, C. Traditional and emerging cardiovascular and renal risk factors: an epidemiological perspective. *Kidney Int.*, 2006, 70(1), 26-33.

[31] Krediet, RT; Balafa, O. Cardiovascular risk in the peritoneal dialysis patient. *Nat Rev Nephrol.*, 2010, 6, 451-460.

[32] Abbott, KC; Glanton, CW; Trespalacios, FC; Oliver, D; Ortiz, MI; Agodoa, LY. Body mass index, dialysis modality, and survival: analysis of the United States Renal Data System Dialysis Morbidity and Mortality Wave ii Study. *Kidney Int.*, 2004, 65, 597-605.

[33] de Mutsert, R; Grootendorst, DC; Boeschoten, EW; Dekker, FW; Krediet, RT. Is obesity associated with a survival advantage in patients starting peritoneal dialysis? *Contrib Nephrol.*, 2009, 163, 124-131.

[34] Lewington, S; Whitlock, G; Clarke, R. Blood cholesterol and vascular mortality by age, sex, and blood pressure: a meta-analysis of individual data from 61 prospective studies with 55,000 vascular deaths. *Lancet.*, 2007, 370, 1829-1839.

[35] Tsimihodimos, V; Mitrogianni, Z; Elisaf, M. Dyslipidemia Associated with Chronic Kidney Disease. *Open Cardiovasc Med J.*, 2011, 5, 41-48.

[36] Anavekar, NS; Solomon, SD; McMurray, JJ; Maggioni, A; Rouelau, JL; Califf, R. Relation between renal dysfunction and cardiovascular outcomes after myocardial infarction. *N Engl J Med.*, 2004, 351, 1285-1295.

[37] Herzig, KA; Purdie, DM; Chang, W; Brown, AM; Hawley, CM; Campbeli, SM. Is C-reactive protein a useful predictor of outcome in peritoneal dialysis patients? *J Am Soc Nephrol.*, 2001, 12, 814-821.

[38] Tatematsu, S; Wakino, S; Kanda, T; Homma, K; Yoshioka, K; Hasegawa, K. Role of nitric oxide producing and -degrading pathways in coronary endothelial dysfunction in chronic kidney disease. *J Am Soc Nephrol.*, 2007, 18, 741-749.

[39] Choi, HY; Lee, JE; Han, SH; Yoo, TH; Kim, BS; Park, HC. Association of inflammation and protein-energy wasting with endothelial dysfunction in peritoneal dialysis patients. *Nephrol Dial Transplant.* 2010, 25, 1266-1271.

[40] Kielstein, JT; Zoccali, C. Asymmetric dimethylarginine: a cardiovascular risk factor and a uremic toxin coming of age? *Am J Kidney Dis.*, 2005, 46, 186-202.

[41] Stenvinkel, P; Heimbürger, O; Paultre, F; Diczfalusy, U; Wang, T; Berglund. L. Strong association between malnutrition, inflammation, and atherosclerosis in chronic renal failure. *Kidney Int.*,1999, 55, 1899-1911.

[42] de Mutsert, R; Grootendorst, DC; Axelsson, J; Boeschoten, EW; Krediet, RT; Dekker, FW. NECOSAD Study Group. Excess mortality due to interaction between protein-energy wasting, inflammation and

cardiovascular disease in chronic dialysis patients. *Nephrol Dial Transplant.*, 2008, 23, 2957-2964.

[43] Chung, SH; Lindholm, B; Lee, HB. Is malnutrition an independent predictor of mortality in peritoneal dialysis patients? *Nephrol Dial Transplant.*, 2003, 18, 2134-2140.

[44] Fouque, D; Kalantar-Zadeh, K; Kopple, J; Cano, N; Chauveau, P; Cuppari, L. A proposed nomenclature and diagnostic criteria for protein-energy wasting in acute and chronic kidney disease. *Kidney Int.*, 2008, 73, 391-398.

[45] de Mutsert, R; Grootendorst, DC; Indemans, F; Boeschoten, EW; Krediet, RT; Dekker, FW. Netherlands Cooperative Study on the Adequacy of Dialysis-II Study Group. Association between serum albumin and mortality in dialysis patients is partly explained by inflammation, and not by malnutrition. *J Ren Nutr.*, 2009, 19, 127-135.

[46] Canada-USA (CANUSA) Peritoneal dialysis Study Group. Adequacy of dialysis and nutrition in continuous peritoneal dialysis: Association with clinical outcomes. *J Am Soc Nephrol.*, 1996, 7, 196-207.

[47] Dounousi, E; Papavasiliou, E; Makedou, A; Ioannou, K; Katopodis, KP; Tselepis, A. Oxidative stress is progressively enhanced with advancing stages of CKD. *Am J Kidney Dis.*, 2006, 48, 752-760.

[48] Ignace, S; Fouque, D; Arkouche, W; Steghens, JP; Guebre-Egziabher, F. Preserved residual renal function is associated with lower oxidative stress in peritoneal dialysis patients. *Nephrol Dial Transplant.*, 2009, 24, 1685-1689.

[49] Boudouris, G; Verginadis, II; Simos, YS; Zouridakis, A; Ragos, V; Karkabounas, SC. Oxidative stress in patients treated with continuous ambulatory peritoneal dialysis (CAPD) and the significant role of vitamin C and E supplementation. *Int Urol Nephrol.*, 2012, 21, 212-216.

[50] Wilson, AM; Kimura, E; Harada, RK; Nair, N; Narasimhan, B; Meng, XY. Beta 2 microglobulin as a biomarker in peripheral arterial disease: proteomic profiling and clinical studies. *Circulation.*, 2009, 116(12), 1396-1403.

[51] Noordzij, M; Korevaar, CJ; Bos, JW; Boeschoten, WE; Dekker, WF; Bossuyt, M. i sur. for the NECOSAD Study Group. Mineral metabolism and cardiovascular morbidity and mortality risk: peritoneal dialysis patients compared with haemodialysis patients. *Nephrol Dial Transplant*, 2006, 21, 2513-2520.

[52] Wang, AY; Wang, M; Woo, J; Lam, CW; Li, PK; Lui, SF. Cardiac valve calcification as an important predictor for all-cause mortality and

cardiovascular mortality in long-term peritoneal dialysis patients: a prospective study. *J Am Soc Nephrol*, 2003, 14, 159-168.

[53]   Wang, AY. Cardiovascular task factors in end-stage renal disease: Beyond Framingham. *Medical Diary.*, 2008, 4, 17-19.

[54]   Haydar, AA; Covic, A; Colhoun, H; Rubens, M; Goldsmith, DJ. Coronary artery calcification and aortic pulse wave velocity in chronic kidney disease patients. *Kidney Int.*, 2004, 65, 1790-1794.

[55]   London, GM; Guérin, AP; Marchais, SJ; Métivier, F; Pannier, B; Adda, H. Arterial media calcification in end-stage renal disease: impact on all-cause and cardiovascular mortality. *Nephrol Dial Transplant.*, 2003, 18, 1731-1740.

[56]   Wang, AY; Woo, J; Lam, CW; Wang, M; Chan, IH; Gao, P. Associations of serum fetuin-A with malnutrition, inflammation, atherosclerosis and valvular calcification syndrome and outcome in peritoneal dialysis patients. *Nephrol Dial Transplant.*, 2005, 20, 1676-1685.

[57]   Shimada, T; Kakitani, M; Yamazaki, Y; Hasegawa, H; Takeuchi, Y; Fujita, T. Targeted ablation of Fgf23 demonstrates an essential physiological role of FGF23 in phosphate and vitamin D metabolism. *J Clin Invest.*, 2004, 113, 561-568.

[58]   Damasiewicz, MJ; Toussaint, ND; Polkinghorne, KR. Fibroblast growth factor 23 in chronic kidney disease: New insights and clinical implications. *Nephrology (Carlton)*, 2011, 16, 261-268.

[59]   Nemcsik, J; Kiss, I; Tisler, A. Arterial stiffness, vascular calcification and bone metabolism in chronic kidney disease. *World J Nephrol.*, 2012, 1(1), 25-34.

[60]   Wang, AY. Serum 25-hydroxyvitamin D status and cardiovascular outcomes in chronic peritoneal dialysis patients: a 3-y prospective cohort study. *Am J Clin Nutr.*, 2008, 87, 1631-1638.

[61]   Suliman, ME; Bárán, YP; Kalantar-Zadeh, K; Lindholm, B; Stenvinkel, P. Homocysteine in uraemia-a puzzling and conflicting story. *Nephrol Dial Transplant.*, 2005, 20, 16-21.

[62]   Suliman, M; Stenvinkel, P; Qureshi, AR; Kalantar-Zadeh, K; Bárány, P; Heimbürger, O. The reverse epidemiology of plasma total homocysteine as a mortality risk factor is related to the impact of wasting and inflammation. *Nephrol Dial Transplant.*, 2007, 22, 209-217.

[63]   Heinz, J; Kropf, S; Domröse, U; Westphal, S; Borucki, K; Luley, C. B vitamins and the risk of total mortality and cardiovascular disease in

endstage renal disease: results of a randomized controlled trial. *Circulation.*, 2010, 30, 1432-1438.

[64] Toshio, O; Taro, M; Nobuyuki, T; Michiva, O; Hiroshi, O. C-reactive protein, lipoprotein(a), homocysteine, and male sex contribute to carotid atherosclerosis in peritoneal dialysis patients. *Am J Kidney Dis.*, 2003, 42(29), 355-361.

[65] Lopez, EG; Carrero, JJ; Suliman, EM; Lindholm, B; Stenvinkel, P. Risk factors for cardiovascular disease in patients undergoing peritoneal dialysis. *Perit Dial Int.*, 2007, 27(S), 205-209.

[66] Fortes, PC; de Moraes, TP; Mendes, JG; Stinghen, AE; Ribeiro, SC; Pecoits-Filho, R. Insulin resistance and glucose homeostasis in peritoneal dialysis. *Perit Dial Int.*, 2009, 29, S145-148.

[67] Rašić, S; Kulenović, I; Zulić, I; Haračić, A; Čengić, M; Unčanin, S. The effect of erythropoietin treatment on left ventricular hypertrophy in haemodialysis patients. *Bosn J Basic Med Sci.*, 2003, 3(4), 11-15.

[68] Singh, AK. Does TREAT give the boot to ESAs in the treatment of CKD anemia? *J Am Soc Nephrol.*, 2010, 21, 2–6.

[69] Pecoits-Filho, R. Managing a Peritoneal Dialysis Patient with High Risk for Cardiovascular Disease. *Nephron Clin Pract.*, 2010, 116, 283-288.

[70] Balafa, O; Krediet, RT. Peritoneal dialysis and cardiovascular disease. *Minerva Urol Nefrol.*, 2012, 64(3), 153-162.

[71] Prinsen, BA. Broad-based metabolic approach to study vLDL apoB-100 metabolism in patients with ESRD and patients with ESRD and patients treated with peritoneal dialysis. *Kidney Int.*, 2004, 65, 1064-1075.

[72] Himmele, R; Savin, DA; Diaz-Buxo, DA. GDPs and AGEs: Impact on cardiovascular toxicity in dialysis patients. *Adv Perit Dial.*, 2011, 27, 22-26.

[73] Williams, JD; Topley, N; Craig, KJ; Mackenzie, RK; Pischetsrieder, M; Lage, C. The Euro-Balance Trial: the effect of a new biocompatible peritoneal dialysis fluid (balance) on the peritoneal membrane. *Kidney Int.*, 2004, 66, 408-418.

[74] Cancarini, GC; Brunori, G; Camerini, I. Renal function recovery and maintenance of residual diuresis in CAPD and haemodialysis. *Perit Dial Int.*, 2002, 6, 77-79.

[75] Smit, W; Schouten, N; van den Berg, N; Langedijk, MJ; Struijk, DG; Krediet, RT. Netherlands Ultrafiltration Failure Study Group. Analysis of the prevalence and causes of ultrafiltration failure during long-term peritoneal dialysis: a cross-sectional study. *Perit. Dial. Int.*, 2004, 24, 562–570.

[76] Bargman, JM; Thorpe, KE; Churchill, DN. Relative contribution of residual renal function and peritoneal clearance to adequacy of dialysis: a reanalysis of the CANUSA study. *J Am Soc Nephrol.*, 2001, 12, 2158-2162.

[77] Paniagua, R; Amato, D; Vonesh, E; Correa-Rotter, R; Ramos, A; Moran, J. Mexican Nephrology Collaborative Study Group. Effects of increased peritoneal clearances on mortality rates in peritoneal dialysis: ADEMEX, a prospective, randomized, controlled trial. *J Am Soc Nephrol.*, 2002, 13, 1307-1320.

[78] Termorshuizen, F; Korevaar, JC; Dekker, FW; van Manen, JG; Boeschoten, EW; Krediet, RT. NECOSAD Study Group.The relative importance of residual renal function compared with peritoneal clearance for patient survival and quality of life: an analysis of the Netherlands Cooperative Study on the Adequacy of Dialysis (NECOSAD)-2. *Am J Kidney Dis.*, 2003, 41, 1293-1302.

[79] Wang, AY; Wang, M; Woo, J. A novel association between residual renal function and left ventricular hypertrophy in peritoneal dialysis patients *Kidney Int.*, 2002, 62, 639–647.

[80] Mallamaci, F; Tripepi, G; Cutrupi, S; Malatino, LS; Zoccali, C. Prognostic value of combined use of biomarkers of inflammation, endothelial dysfunction, and myocardiopathy in patients with ESRD. *Kidney Int.*, 2005, 67, 2330–2337.

[81] Rutten, JH; Korevaar, JC; Boeschoten, EW; Dekker, FW; Krediet, RT; Boomsma, F; van den Meiracker, AH. B-type natriuretic peptide and amino-terminal atrial natriuretic peptide predict survival in peritoneal dialysis. *Perit. Dial. Int.*, 2006, 26, 598-602.

[82] Wang, AY; Lam, CW; Yu, CM; Wang, M; Chan, IH; Zhang, Y. N-terminal pro-brain natriuretic peptide: an independent risk predictor of cardiovascular congestion, mortality, and adverse cardiovascular outcomes in chronic peritoneal dialysis patients. *J Am Soc Nephrol.*, 2007, 18, 321–330.

[83] Krediet, RT. Dry body weight: water and sodium removal targets in PD. *Contrib Nephrol.*, 2006, 150, 104-110.

[84] Balakrishnan, VS; Guo, D; Rao, M; Jaberm, BL; Tighiouart, H; Freeman, RL. Cytokine gene polymorphisms in hemodialysis patients: association with comorbidity, functionality, and serum albumin. *Kidney Int.*, 2004, 65, 1449-1460.

[85] Losito, A; Kalidas, K; Santoni, S; Jeffery, S. Association of interleukin-6-174G/C promoter polymorphism with hypertension and left

ventricular hypertrophy in dialysis patients. *Kidney Int.*, 2003, 64, 616 - 622.

[86] Lang, RM; Bierig, M; Devereux, RB; Flaschskampf, FA; Foster, E; Pellikka, PA. Recommendations for chamber quantification: a report from the American Society of Echocardiography's Guidelines and Standards Committee and the Chamber Quantification Writing Group, developed in conjunction with the European Association of Echocardiography, a branch of the European Society of Cardiology. *J Am Soc Echocardiogr.*, 2005, 18, 1440–1463.

[87] Chung, SH; Chu, WS; Lee, HA; Kim, YH; Lee, IS; Lindholm, B; Lee, HB. Peritoneal transport characteristics, comorbid diseases and survival in CAPD patients. *Perit Dial Int.*, 2000, 20, 541–547.

[88] Coll, B; Betriu, A; Alonso, MM; Borras, M; Craver, L; Amoedo, LM; Marco, MP; Sarro, F; Junyent, M; Valdivielso, JM; Fernandez, E. Cardiovascular risk factors underestimate atherosclerotic burden in chronic kidney disease: usefulness of non-invasive tests in cardiovascular assessment. *Nephrol Dial Transplant.*, 2010, 25, 3017–3025.

[89] Akcay, A; Ozdemir, FN; Sezer, S; Micozkadioglu, H; Arat, Z; Atac, FB. Association of vitamin D receptor gene polymorphisms with hypercalcemia in peritoneal dialysis patients. *Perit Dial Int.*, 2005, 25(3), S52 -S55.

[90] Stenvinkel, P; Karimi, M; Johansson, S; Axelsson, J; Suliman, M; Lindholm, B. Impact of inflammation on epigenetic DNA methylation-a novel risk factor for cardiovascular disease? *JIntern Med.*, 2007, 261, 488-499.

[91] Devereux, R; Alonso, D; Lutas, E; Gottlieb, G; Compo, E; Reichek, N. Echocardiographic assessment of left ventricular hypertrophy: comparison to necropsy findings. *Am J Cardiol.*, 1986, 57, 450-458.

[92] Devereux, RB; Reichek, N. Echocardiographic determination of left ventricular mass in man. Anatomic validation of the method. *Circulation*, 1977, 55, 613–618.

[93] Szeto, CC; Chow, KM; Woo, KS; Chook, P; Kwan, HC; Leung, BC. Carotid Intima Media Thickness Predicts Cardiovascular Diseases in Chinese Predialysis Patients with Chronic Kidney Disease. *J Am Soc Nephrol.*,2007, 18(6), 1966-1972.

[94] Coll, B; Betriu, A; Alonso, MM; Borràs, M; Craver, L; Amoedo, ML. Cardiovascular risk factors underestimate atherosclerotic burden in chronic kidney disease: usefulness of non-invasive tests in

cardiovascular assessment. *Nephrol Dial Transplant.*, 2010, 25(9), 3017-3025.

[95] Junyent, M; Gilabert, R; Núñez, I; Corbella, E; Vela, M; Zambón, D. Carotid ultrasound in the assessment of preclinical atherosclerosis. Distribution of intima–media thickness values and plaque frequency in a Spanish community cohort. *Med Clin (Barc).*, 2005, 125, 770-774.

[96] Caliskan, Y; Ozkok, A; Akagun, T; Alpay, N; Guz, G; Polat, N. Cardiac Biomarkers and Noninvasive Predictors of Atherosclerosis in Chronic Peritoneal Dialysis Patients. *Kidney Blood Press Res.*, 2012, 35, 340-348.

[97] Locatelli, F; Pozzoni, P; Tentori, F; del Vecchio, L. Epidemiology of cardiovascular risk in patients with chronic kidney disease. *Nephrol Dial Transplant.*, 2003, 18(7), 2-9.

[98] Benedetto, AF; Tripepi, G; Mallamaci, F; Zoccali, C. Rate of atherosclerotic plaque formation predicts cardiovascular events in ESRD. *J Am Soc Nephrol.*, 2008, 19(4), 757-763.

[99] de Jager, DJ; Grootendorst, DC; Jager, KJ; van Dijk, PC; Tomas, LM; Ansell, D. Cardiovascular and noncardiovascular mortality among patients starting dialysis. *JAMA.*, 2009, 302, 1782-1789.

[100] Parfrey, PS; Foley, RN; Harnett, JD; Kent, GM; Murray, D; Barre, PE. Outcome and risk factors of ischemic heart disease in chronic uremia. *Kidney Int.*, 1996, 49, 1428-1434.

[101] Wang, AY. Vascular and other tissue calcification in peritoneal dialysis patients. *Perit Dial Int.*, 2009, 29(2), S9-S14.

[102] Blacher, J; Pannier, B; Guerin, AP; Marchais, SJ; Safar, ME; London, GM. Carotid arterial stiffness as a predictor of cardiovascular and all-cause mortality in end stage renal disease. *Hypertension*, 1998, 32, 570-574.

[103] K/DOQI Clinical Practice Guidelines for Cardiovascular Disease in Dialysis. *Am J Kidney Dis.*, 2005, 45, S1-153.

[104] Stompor, T; Krasniak, A; Sulowicz, W; Kieć, DA; Janda, K; Wojcik, K. Changes in common carotid artery intima-media thickness over 1-year in patients on peritoneal dialysis. *Nephrol Dial Transplant.*, 2005, 20 (2), 404-412.

[105] Schalkwijk, CG; Stehouwer, CD. Vascular complications in diabetes mellitus: the role of endothelial dysfunction. *Clin Sci.*, 2005, 109, 143-159.

[106] Mutluay, R; Degertekin, CK; Poyraz, F; Yilmaz, MI; Yucel, C; Turfan, M. Dialysis type may predict carotid intima media thickness and plaque

presence in end-stage renal disease patients. *Adv Ther.*, 2012, 29(4), 370-382.

[107] Chiu, YW; Mehrotra, R. Can we reduce the cardiovascular risk in peritoneal dialysis patients? *Indian J Nephrol.*, 2010, 20, 59-67.

[108] Cengiz, K; Dolu, D. Comparison of atherosclerosis and atherosclerotic risk factors in patients receiving hemodialysis and peritoneal dialysis. *Dial Transplant.*, 2007, 36, 205-216.

[109] Mancia, G; Fagard, R; Narkiewicz, K; Redan, J; Zanchetti, A; Bohm, M. 2013 ESH/ESC Guidelines for the management of arterial hypertension. *J Hypertens.*, 2013, 31(10), 1925-38.

[110] Levin, A; Rigatto, C; Brendan, B; Madore, F; Muirhead, N; Holmes, D. Cohort profile:Canadian study of prediction of death,dialysis and interim cardiovascular events (CanPREDDICT). *BMC Nephrol.*, 2013, 14, 121. doi:10.1186/1471-2369-14-121.

[111] Tonbul, Z; Altintepe, L; Sözlü, C; Yeksan, M; Yildiz, A; Türk, S. Ambulatory blood pressure monitoring in haemodialysis and continuous ambulatory peritoneal dialysis (CAPD) patients. *J Hum Hypertens.*,2002, 16(8), 585-589.

[112] Lewington, S; Whitlock, G; Clarke, R; Sherliker, P; Emberson, J; Halsey, J. Blood cholesterol and vascular mortality by age, sex, and blood pressure: a meta-analysis of individual data from 61 prospective studies with 55, 000 vascular deaths. *Lancet.*,2007, 370, 1829-1839.

[113] Longenecker, CJ; Coresh, J; Powe, RN; Levey, SA; Fink, EN; Martin, A. Traditional Cardiovascular Disease Risk Factors in Dialysis Patients Compared with the General Population: The CHOICE Study. *J Am Soc Nephrol.*,2002, 13 (7), 1918-1927.

[114] Despres, JP; Lemieux, I; Dagenais, GR; Cantin, B; Lamarche, B. HDL-cholesterol as a marker of coronary heart disease risk: the Quebec cardiovascular study. *Atherosclerosis.*, 2000, 153, 263-272.

[115] Cengiz, K; Dolu, D. Comparison of atherosclerosis and atherosclerotic risk factors in patients receiving hemodialysis and peritoneal dialysis. *Dial Transplant.*, 2007, 36, 205-216.

[116] Wang, AY; Woo, J; Lam, CW; Wang, M; Sea, MM; Lui, SF. Is a single time point C-reactive protein predictive of outcome in peritoneal dialysis patients? *J Am Soc Nephrol.*, 2003, 14, 1871-1879.

[117] Termorshuizen, F; Korevaar, JC; Dekker, FW; van Manen, JG; Boeschoten, EW; Krediet, RT. NECOSAD Study Group.The relative importance of residual renal function compared with peritoneal clearance for patient survival and quality of life: an analysis of the

Netherlands Cooperative Study on the Adequacy of Dialysis (NECOSAD)-2. *Am J Kidney Dis.*, 2003, 41, 1293-1302.

[118] Mizobuchi, M; Towler, D; Slatopolsky, E. Vascular calcification: the killer of patients with chronic kidney disease. *J Am Soc Nephrol.*, 2009, 20, 1453-1464.

[119] Wang, AY; Woo, J; Lam, CW; Wang, M; Sea, MM; Lui, SF. Is a single time point C-reactive protein predictive of outcome in peritoneal dialysis patients? *J Am Soc Nephrol.*, 2003, 14, 1871-1879.

[120] Paniagua, R; Amato, D; Mujais, S; Vonesh, E; Ramos, A; Correa-Rotter, R; Horl, WH. Predictive value of brain natriuretic peptides in patients on peritoneal dialysis: results from the ADEMEX trial. *Clin J Am Soc Nephrol.*, 2008, 3, 407–415.

[121] Rašić, S; Kulenović, I; Haračić, A; Ćatović, A. Left ventricular hypertrophy and risk factors for its development in uraemic patients. *Bosn J Basic Med Sci.*, 2004, 4(1), 34-40.

[122] Huang, CH; Chang, CC; Chang, TL; Chang, YJ. Dynamic cardiac dyssynchrony is strongly associated with 2-year dialysis adequacy in continuous ambulatory peritoneal dialysis patients. *BMC Nephrol.*,2013, 23, 14, 68. doi: 10.1186/1471-2369-14-68.

In: Cardiac Remodeling
Editor: Jerald Sherman

ISBN: 978-1-63484-270-9
© 2016 Nova Science Publishers, Inc.

Chapter 2

TROPOMYOSIN:
AN EFFECTOR OF CARDIAC REMODELING

David F. Wieczorek[*]
Department of Molecular Genetics, Biochemistry, and Microbiology
University of Cincinnati Medical Center, Cincinnati, Ohio, US

ABSTRACT

Tropomyosin (Tpm), an α-helical coiled coil protein, is an integral component of the thin filament in the cardiac muscle sarcomere. Striated muscle contraction is regulated through a calcium (Ca^{2+}) –dependent mechanism involving Tpm, troponin, actin, and myosin. Tpm occupies a unique structural position by serving as the intermediary effector that repositions itself when Ca^{2+} binds troponin. When Ca^{2+} binds to troponin C, a conformational change occurs allowing Tpm to shift its position and move away from the myosin binding sites on the sarcomeric actin filament, resulting in the myosin head binding to actin and leading to muscle contraction. There are three primary striated muscle Tpm isoforms generated from distinct genes. Our laboratory has focused on understanding the function of these Tpm isoforms. Studies from our laboratory demonstrate that increased expression of the embryonic cardiac β-Tpm isoform can lead to a dramatic hypertrophic cardiomyopathic condition. In addition, mutations in Tpm are associated with human hypertrophic (HCM) and dilated (DCM) cardiomyopathies.

---

[*] Email: david.wieczorek@uc.edu.

In order to investigate HCM and DCM conditions caused by Tpm mutations, we generated animal models that incorporate these HCM and DCM mutations. An advantage in using transgenic mice is that the endogenous α-Tpm isoform decreases its expression in proportion with increased expression of exogenous Tpm expression through both post-transcriptional and translational regulatory mechanisms. We find incorporation of these HCM- and DCM-causing Tpm mutations in transgenic mice lead to cardiac remodeling that resembles the pathological changes found in hypertrophic or dilated cardiomyopathy patients; in addition, physiological alterations also occur in the diseased murine myocardium that reflect the functional abnormalities found in HCM and DCM patients. Furthermore, we found that modulation of the phosphorylation status of Tpm can also trigger cardiac remodeling . Interestingly, our studies show the aberrant phenotypes that are generated by Tpm mutations can also be "rescued" through modifications in Tpm which affect the myofilament's response to Ca^{2+}. These studies demonstrate that Tpm plays a unique role in its ability to not only cause morphological and functional alterations in the diseased heart, but it can also reverse the pathological and physiological remodeling that occurs during cardiomyopathic conditions.

INTRODUCTION

Tropomyosin (Tpm) is an essential protein that plays multiple roles within cells and tissues. In non-muscle cells, Tpm is associated with actin and the microtubules, contributing to the cytoskeletal architecture of the cell. It also functions in essential processes, such as cytokinesis and axoplasmic transport. In smooth muscle cells, Tpm functions in muscle contraction through its association with actin and myosin. Although much is known about Tpm in non-muscle and smooth muscle cells, its role in the thin filament of striated muscle has been extensively investigated. The focus of this review is on the role of the different Tpm striated muscle isoforms, their function, and the response in cardiac remodeling that occurs with various mutations and alterations in phosphorylation status. Throughout this review, we will cite specific examples of how specific mutations and modifications to Tpm trigger a physiological, hypertrophic, or dilated cardiomyopathic remodeling response, oftentimes associated with the response of the myofilament to calcium. Cardiac remodeling has been defined as changes in genomic expression, and alterations in molecular, cellular, and interstitial processes that are manifest as changes in size, shape and function of the heart following physiological or pathological conditions [1, 2]. The cardiomyocyte is the primary cell involved in the remodeling process, but other components include the interstitium, fibroblasts, and the vasculature. In this review, we will also cite examples where modifications in Tpm expression or phosphorylation can "rescue" a cardiomyopathic condition resulting in a normal morphological and physiological phenotype.

TROPOMYOSIN STRUCTURE AND FUNCTION

Tpm is encoded in by 4 distinct genes (1, 2, 3, and 4 (alternatively named α, β, γ, and δ, respectively), each of which undergoes alternative splicing to generate multiple mRNA and protein isoforms. Each of these genes is presumed to have evolved from a common ancestral gene, with expression of Tpm being found in yeast (*S. cerevisiae* and *S. pombe*) through humans [3]. The high degree of nucleotide and amino acid sequence conservation has led to individual genes and proteins that are very similar in their basic structure. The basic structure of the Tpm protein is a dimeric coiled-coil α-helical structure of either 248 or 284 amino acids. The two chains associate in parallel and in register to make a rod-shaped molecule that binds along the grooves of the helical actin filament [4].

Tpm's primary function is to bind to the actin filament. This binding occurs with cytoplasmic, smooth muscle, and striated muscle actin depending upon the specific Tpm isoform and its function within the cell. During embryonic stem cell differentiation and early stages of murine embryogenesis, multiple Tpm isoforms are expressed from all 4 of the genes [5]. Many cells, such as neurons and muscle cells, express these multiple Tpm isoforms simultaneously, and these isoforms change dependent upon the developmental stage and physiological function of the particular cell or tissue. For example, in neurons, Tpm isoforms are associated with growth cones, axoplasmic transport, and cytoskeletal architecture. In striated muscle, Tpm is associated with the cytoskeletal architecture and with the thin filament of the sarcomere; during the transition from myoblasts to myotubes, the ratio of cytoskeletal to striated muscle Tpm isoforms decreases during muscle differentiation. Although this ratio changes with muscle differentiation, there appears to always be at least 20% cytoskeletal Tpm in differentiated striated muscle [6]. The simultaneous expression of multiple Tpm isoforms attests to their diverse functions within specific cells and tissues.

As mentioned, in skeletal and cardiac muscle, Tpm is associated with the thin filament of the sarcomere and plays an active role in the regulation of contraction. In the thin filament, Tpm binds to both actin and the troponin (Tn) complex which consists of TnT, TnI and TnC. In the relaxation state, Tpm binds to actin and blocks the myosin head binding sites on actin. When calcium (Ca^{2+}) binds to TnC, changes in the Tn complex imparts a repositioning of Tpm on the actin filament which exposes the myosin binding sites, resulting in the myosin head binding to actin and leading to muscle contraction. There is also movement of both TnT and TnI with Ca^{2+} binding to TnC. When Ca^{2+} releases from TnC and is re-sequestered into the sarcoplasmic reticulum, Tpm resumes its blocking position on the thin filament resulting in sarcomeric relaxation.

TPM ISOFORM EXPRESSION IN STRIATED MUSCLE

The expression of Tpm in skeletal muscle is complex due to the diversity of muscle types: fast glycolytic, fast oxidative, and slow oxidative. In addition, there are 3 principle Tpm striated muscle isoforms that are expressed in skeletal muscle: Tpm1 skα, Tpm2 skβ, and Tpm3 skγ. Each of these isoforms is highly homologous in their amino acid sequences: Tpm1 skα demonstrates an 87% identity with Tpm2 skβ, and a 91% identity with Tpm3 skγ [7]. Each muscle appears to express at least two of these isoforms [8, 9]. Fast glycolytic and fast oxidative muscles primarily express skα and skβ; slow twitch muscle express 45% of skα, 25 – 30% of skβ, and 25-30% skγ. During development, embryonic and newborn skeletal muscle express approximately 60% skβ and 35% skα, with low levels of skγ. As previously stated, when adult skeletal muscle differentiates into complex muscle fibers, the expression of the Tpm isoforms correlates with the speed and metabolic properties of the muscle. In extraocular muscles which possess fast glycolytic, fast oxidative, slow oxidative, and slow tonic fibers, Tpm expression appears to be restricted to skα and skβ isoforms, although a more comprehensive analysis needs to be conducted [10, 11]. In the heart, skα and skβ are the predominant isoforms that are expressed; from the early stages of cardiac morphogenesis through the adult stage, the α/β striated muscle Tpm isoform ratio increases from 4 – 60, making skα the predominant isoform in the adult heart [5]. There is also a minor Tpm striated muscle isoform (α-Tpmκ) expressed in axolotl, chicken, and human hearts [12-14].

TPM ISOFORM KNOCKOUTS AND OVEREXPRESSION IN MICE

The essential nature of Tpm in striated muscle has been demonstrated through knockout strategies of the Tpm isoforms. Knocking out the Tpm1 isoform in the mouse leads to lethality in the developing mouse embryo between 8-11.5 days p.c. [15, 16]. This lethal event corresponds to the developmental period of cardiogenesis, strongly suggestive that Tpm1 plays an essential role for sarcomeric function that cannot be substituted for with other Tpm isoforms. This idea is strengthened by the fact that in heterozygous knockout Tpm1 mice with a 50% reduction in skα mRNA levels, a translational mechanism is activated so that normal amounts of protein are produced and incorporated into the myofibril; this translational mechanism is accomplished by increasing the number of polyribosomes on the Tpm1 skα mRNA [16]. Knocking out the Tpm3 gene is also a lethal event; however, this knockout results in the inability of the fertilized egg to implant during embryogenesis [17]. This also demonstrates the essential nature of Tpm for implantation and survival of the developing embryo. A knockout of Tpm2 also appears to be an early lethal event, similar to the Tpm 3 knockout, although this observation needs further exploration (Rajan and Wieczorek, unpublished results). Collectively, the results from the Tpm knockout studies demonstrate the essential nature of Tpm for both implantation and maturation of the developing embryo. This fact is also supported by the fact that isoforms of these 3 genes are expressed during the earliest stages of embryogenesis [5]. Also, it is interesting that with the knockout studies, that despite the high degree of amino acid similarity that exists among the Tpm isoforms, substitution by the other Tpm genes and isoforms cannot compensate for the ablated genes, thus demonstrating the essential nature of each of these genes and their associated isoforms.

Although the Tpm2 and Tpm3 knockout studies result in failure of implantation, the Tpm1 knockout mice develop until 8-11 days p.c. With this survival, it is interesting to note that there is no gross evidence of remodeling in the developing embryo, including the heart. This is not the case in studies investigating Tpm isoform overexpression. When Tpm2 skβ is overexpressed in the hearts of transgenic mice, there are molecular and physiological changes that compensate for this altered isoform expression. This level of expression was a 150-fold increase in mRNA expression, with a 34-fold increase in the associated protein [18]. On the molecular level, this increased expression of the Tpm2 skβ transgene also leads to a reciprocal decrease in the levels of Tpm1 skα transcripts and its associated protein which results in no net change in total Tpm levels. There are no detectable alterations in the expression of other contractile protein genes, including the endogenous Tpm2 isoforms [18, 19]. Physiologically, these transgenic hearts exhibit a significant decrease in the rate of relaxation with an associated increase in the time of one-half relaxation (Table 1). There is also a significant increase in Ca^{2+} sensitivity of the myofilaments [19], along with decreased maximum tension and ATPase activity in the extracted transgenic cardiac myofibers [20]. Interestingly, there are no structural changes observed in these transgenic hearts with this level of transgene expression. However, when Tpm2 skβ is expressed in transgenic mouse hearts at higher levels (i.e., 75-80% skβ expression), there is significant cardiac remodeling that results in dramatic atrial and ventricular enlargement, coupled with thrombus formation in the lumen of the cardiac chambers, fibrosis, and diffuse myocytolysis [21]. Both contractile and relaxation parameters are severely impaired and these mice die between 10-14 days postpartum. These results firmly demonstrate essential differences in Tpm isoform function in physiologically regulating cardiac performance.

As stated previously, there is 87% amino acid identity between Tpm1 skα and Tpm2 skβ proteins. To define whether the Tpm regions that bind troponin T play an integral role in the functional differences between skα and skβ, in a series of investigations, we exchanged these regions and examined their physiological effects on cardiac and myofilament function [7, 22-24]. Studies show that troponin T binds to Tpm in two distinct regions: at the carboxyl end of the molecule (amino acids 258-284) , and internally in the region of amino acids 175-190 [25, 26]. When the carboxyl terminal region of skα was substituted with skβ, there were no morphological alterations in the heart, but there were significant functional changes. Physiological alterations included decreases in the rates of cardiac contraction and relaxation, concomitant with increases in the time to peak pressure and end diastolic pressure [22]. There was also a significant decrease in myofilament Ca^{2+} sensitivity.

When the internal troponin T binding region in Tpm1 skα (amino acids 175–190) was exchanged for Tpm2 skβ, there were no pathological differences in these transgenic hearts [24]. However, there were decreases in the maximum rates of contraction and relaxation, coupled with a significant increase in myofilament Ca^{2+} sensitivity. These results demonstrate that the putative internal troponin T binding domain of Tpm can increase Ca^{2+} sensitivity of the thin filament and affect sarcomeric performance at the myofilament level which culminates in altered function at the whole heart level.

Table 1. Comparison of cardiac and sarcomeric morphological and physiological parameters in various transgenic mouse models with respect to α-Tpm (NTG) hearts

Mouse Model	Phenotype	Physiological Parameters		
		Systolic Function	Diastolic Function	Myofilament Ca^{2+} Sensitivity
α-Tm	–	100%	100%	100%
β-Tm	HCM with ↑↑ exp.	–	↓	↑
γ-Tm	–	↑	↑	↓
Tpm 180	HCM	–	↓	↑
Tpm 175	HCM	↓	↓	↑
Tpm 54	DCM	↓	↓	↓
Tpm κ	DCM	↓	↓	↓
Tpm S283A	Physiol.	–	–	–
Tpm S283D	DCM	–	↓	–

To test whether both troponin T binding regions in Tpm might act synergistically to attain normal myofilament Ca^{2+} sensitivity, we generated transgenic mice that simultaneously switched both regions of Tpm1 skα with Tpm2 skβ [23]. Results show that similar to other chimeric Tpm transgenic models, there are abnormalities in cardiac performance, specifically with decreases in their rates of contraction and relaxation, without observable alterations in cardiac morphology. However, there are no differences in myofilament Ca^{2+} sensitivity when compared with littermate control hearts. Our hypothesis for this observation is that both TnT binding regions in Tpm must act synergistically to normalize myofilament Ca^{2+} sensitivity [7].

Under normal conditions, Tpm3 skγ is not expressed in the heart. When Tpm3 skγ is expressed in transgenic hearts, the mice exhibit normal life spans with no signs of cardiac remodeling or morphological abnormalities in their sarcomeres or hearts [27]. Physiological assessment of these mice reveals a hyperdynamic effect on systolic and diastolic function (Table 1). Cardiac myofiber analyses demonstrate a decreased sensitivity to Ca^{2+} in force generation and a decrease in length-dependent Ca^{2+} activation. Similar to the Tpm2 skβ mouse hearts, these transgenic mice also decrease the endogenous expression of Tpm1 skα in response to the transgenic expression of skγ so that the total amount of Tpm is unchanged in the cardiac myocytes.

Studies were conducted to determine the effect of simultaneous expression of all 3 striated muscle Tpm isoforms on cardiac performance. Transgenic mice were generated that expressed Tpm1 skα, Tpm2 skβ, and Tpm3 skγ in equivalent amounts in the heart [7]. Results show these double transgenic hearts do not develop pathological abnormalities; however, they exhibit a hyper contractile phenotype with decreased myofilament Ca^{2+} sensitivity, similar to the Tpm3 skγ transgenic cardiac myofilaments. Thus, there appears to be a functional dominance of Tpm3 skγ over Tpm1 skα or Tpm2 skβ in the regulation of physiological performance of the cardiac muscle sarcomere.

INVOLVEMENT OF TPM IN CARDIAC REMODELING HYPERTROPHY

The association of sarcomeric contractile proteins in human cardiac disease was first demonstrated by Drs. J. and C. Seidman who published in 1990 that missense mutations in myosin heavy chain correlated with familial hypertrophic cardiomyopathy [28]. The association of Tpm with hypertrophic cardiomyopathy (HCM) was initially reported by the Seidman laboratory in 1993 [29, 30]. HCM is an autosomal dominant disease characterized by hypertrophy in the left ventricle and interventricular septum, resulting in a decreased left ventricle volume. Obstruction of the left ventricular outflow tract is present in ~25% of patients [31]. There is often myocyte disarray and interstitial fibrosis, coupled with systolic hypercontractility and impaired relaxation and increased myofilament sensitivity to Ca^{2+}. These functional abnormalities can cause progressive heart failure and sudden cardiac death. In the United States, the association of patients with mutations in Tpm causing HCM is relatively few, accounting for less than 5% of all cases [32]. Although the incidence of HCM due to Tpm mutations is similar in the Japanese population, the pathological symptoms are much more severe than those found in patients in the United States [33, 34]. However, in Finland, Tpm associated cases are the most prevalent of all the contractile proteins involved in causing HCM; this is most likely due to a 'founder's effect [35]. The pathology of the disease in the Finnish population is quite severe with a majority of patients exhibiting a dramatic phenotype. The variability of the incidence and the pathology associated with Tpm-induced HCM in the different populations most likely reflects environmental influences and modifier genes in altering the onset and phenotype of HCM.

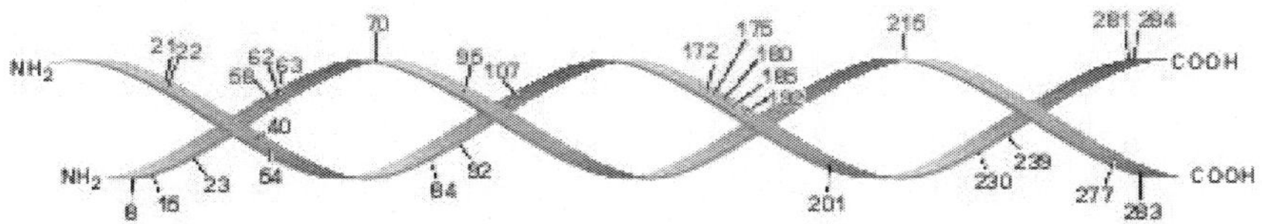

Figure 1. Mutations in α-tropomyosin that are linked to cardiovascular disease. Diagramed in the figure is the Tpm1 skα dimer. The numbers above the Tpm dimer shown in red represent the amino acid residues where mutations have been found that cause HCM (hypertrophic cardiomyopathy). The numbers below the Tpm dimer shown in blue represent where mutations have been found associated with DCM (dilated cardiomyopathy).

Sixteen mutational sites have been found in Tpm1 that lead to HCM (Figure 1) [31]. Each of these mutations is a missense mutation causing a single amino acid substitution, and no truncation or nonsense mutations have been reported. There does not appear to be any consistent pattern for the HCM mutations to be associated with a specific actin-binding repeat, TnT binding region, or a specific residue within the heptad repeat of Tpm. However, a constant feature of HCM mutations that have been tested is that most Tpm mutations increase myofilament Ca^{2+} sensitivity. Nevertheless, due to the diversity of the HCM mutations with the Tpm1 gene, the precise mechanism(s) that is/are activated to cause the HCM phenotype are unknown and may, if fact, differ among the mutations.

Studies of HCM patients by Bottinelli et al. [36] carrying the Asp175Asn Tpm1 mutation found that its expression most likely contributes to the alterations observed in sarcomeric performance, rather than a null allele or a decreased amount of total Tpm. Also, the myofibers from these patients exhibit an increased sensitivity to Ca^{2+} when compared to control fibers. In an attempt to understand the process and pathways that are activated by mutations in Tpm1 that result in an HCM phenotype, we generated transgenic mouse models of the Asp175Asn HCM mutation [37]. Results demonstrate that the Asp175Asn mutation caused a mild cardiac remodeling phenotype in transgenic mouse hearts with hypertrophy, patchy areas of myocyte disorganization, occasional thrombi formation in the left atria, severe fibrosis, and atrial thrombi and mineralization. Physiological analyses demonstrated the diseased hearts exhibited severe impairment of both contractility and relaxation, with an increased activation of the thin filament through enhanced

Ca^{2+} sensitivity of steady-state force (Table 1) [37, 38]. Studies also show that HCM patients with the Asp175Asn mutation exhibit a significantly increased Ca^{2+} sensitivity of force generation in skinned fiber preparations [36]. HCM patients are also susceptible to life-threatening episodes with strenuous exercise. When the Asp175Asn transgenic mice were subject to 8 weeks of swimming exercise, there was a slight increase in fibrosis and myocyte disarray, but no substantial change in viability or degree of hypertrophy. Interestingly, a transgenic Asp175Asn rat HCM model displayed a decreased sensitivity to Ca^{2+} in the myofilaments [39].

As mentioned previously, human patients with this mutation exhibit a mild hypertrophic phenotype in the United States, but a more dramatic phenotype in other populations. To further examine the molecular and physiological mechanisms underlying HCM associated with Tpm mutations, we generated transgenic mice incorporating the Glu180Gly HCM mutation in Tpm1 [40]. Results show the hearts from these mice develop severe concentric hypertrophy, fibrosis and atrial enlargement, with initial pathological changes visible by 1 month and death often occurring between 5-6 months. Both the rates of contraction and relaxation in these hearts are severely impaired, coupled with an increased activation of the thin filament through enhanced calcium sensitivity of steady-state force (Table 1) [40, 41]. Isolated cardiomyocytes from the transgenic mouse hearts also exhibit an increase in calcium sensitivity of force production [42], thus demonstrating that individual myocytes collectively cause the aberrant function of the entire heart leading to cardiac remodeling and hypertrophy. In vitro studies show that the Glu180Gly protein binds much weaker to actin than wild type or Asp175Asn proteins, an observation supported by structural analyses [43-45].

One interesting fact is that the FHC mutations which are autosomal dominant cause dramatic cardiac remodeling to occur, yet there is minimal effect on skeletal muscle morphology or function. There may be multiple reasons for this occurrence. Tpm expression in the heart primarily occurs as Tpm1 skα homodimers, whereas in skeletal muscle, all 3 Tpm isoforms (α-, β-, and γ-Tpm) are expressed. This expression of multiple Tpm isoforms leads to a heterogenous mixture of Tpm homo- and heterodimers that potentially could compensate for mutations in the Tpm1 isoform. Another possibility for the minimal effects of HCM mutations in skeletal muscle is the diversity of expression of the sarcomeric proteins in skeletal muscle, particularly with thick and thin myofilament proteins expressing both fast and slow skeletal isoforms (i.e., TnT, TnI, myosin heavy chain). Thus, the activation of the cardiac remodeling phenotype associated with HCM Tpm mutations, yet without complementary morphological changes occurring in skeletal musculature appears to due to Tpm dimer formation, increased diversity of sarcomeric protein expression, including Tpm, and other differentiating features that exist between cardiac and skeletal musculature.

RESCUE OF THE HCM PHENOTYPE

With the development of gene therapy, researchers have explored ways to "rescue" the hypertrophic cardiomyopathy phenotype through the expression of various transgenes. For HCM, these transgenes express proteins that often modify calcium cycling through direct or indirect mechanisms. With the HCM α-Tpm180 model, we have taken several different approaches. In an attempt to normalize Ca^{2+} sensitivity of the cardiac myofilaments, we generated mice that expressed a chimeric α-/β-Tpm protein in the hearts of these HCM mice [46]. The rationale behind these experiments was that the chimeric α-/β-Tpm protein being exogenously expressed results in decreased sensitivity to Ca^{2+} exhibited by myofilaments. By genetically crossing α-Tpm180 mice with these chimeric α-/β-Tpm mice, we hoped to normalize myofilament Ca^{2+} sensitivity and prevent the development of the HCM phenotype. Results show these double transgenic mice exhibited a normal morphology with no signs of pathological cardiac remodeling. Physiological analyses showed improved cardiac function and normal myofilament Ca^{2+} sensitivity. This study demonstrates that alterations in myofilament Ca^{2+} sensitivity by modification of contractile proteins can prevent the pathological and physiological effects of this disease.

Experiments were employed that directly determined whether modifications to Ca^{2+} handling could rescue the hypertrophic phenotype in the α-Tpm180 mice. The sarcoplasmic reticulum Ca^{2+} ATPase (Serca2a) is responsible for the incorporation of cytosolic Ca^{2+} into the sarcoplasmic reticulum (SR) in cardiomyocytes. In a series of experiments, Serca2a was injected into the left ventricle of control and α-Tpm180 neonates with adenoviral expression vectors to test whether it was possible to delay/prevent the development of hypertrophy and improve cardiac function with increased levels of Serca2a [47]. Results show that delivery of a single dose of Serca2a in 1-day-old mice is sufficient to alter hypertrophic gene expression and improve cardiac morphology. Additional studies show that delivery of Serca2a into experimental models of heart failure in sheep and swine can largely

                    David F. Wieczorek

reverse cardiac dysfunction and improve systolic and diastolic performance in the heart [48, 49]. More recently, heart failure patients have been administered adeno-associated virus expressing Serca2a, and they show marked improvement in ejection fraction and end-systolic dimensions [50, 51]. These results illustrate the potential of using Serca2a-mediated gene transfer as a possible therapy for HCM and/or heart failure patients.

In a complementary study, Gaffin et al. [52] examined whether ablation of phospholamban (PLN) could rescue the α-Tpm180 cardiac HCM phenotype in mice. PLN is the regulator of Serca2a activity in the uptake of Ca^{2+} from the cytosol into the SR. The rationale behind these experiments was that by removing the inhibitory PLN regulator from the SR, Ca^{2+} uptake would be increased by endogenous Serca2a. Results demonstrate that the PLN knock-out/α-Tpm180 mice exhibited normal cardiac physiological function and improved heart morphology, thus reversing the cardiac remodeling that occurs in the α-Tpm180 hearts alone. Additional microarray analyses on the PLN knock-out/α-Tpm180 hearts identified the most significant 62 genes involved in suppression of the HCM phenotype [53]; many of these genes are associated with cardiac hypertrophy, the vasculature, and/or inflammation.

During the course of examining the α-Tpm180 transgenic mice, we assayed the level of Tpm phosphorylation at 3 months, a time when the transgenic hearts have undergone substantial cardiac remodeling to become hypertrophic. Tpm is phosphorylated at a single site: Ser283, the penultimate amino acid of the protein. Results show that at 3 months of age during which time there is significant cardiac pathology, the level of Tpm phosphorylation is significantly higher than wild type levels [54]. Surprisingly, when the α-Tpm180 transgenic mice are crossed with a mouse that does not have the ability to phosphorylate α-Tpm (α-Tpm S283A), the HCM phenotype is rescued [54]. These double mutant transgenic mice (α-Tpm 180/α-Tpm S283A) exhibit no signs of cardiac hypertrophy and display improved cardiac function. The myofilaments from the double transgenic mice do show an increased Ca^{2+} sensitivity compared with wild type controls, but this is still significantly less than the sensitivity exhibited by α-Tpm180 myofilaments. There were no changes in Serca2a gene or protein expression, but there was an increase in phosphorylation of PLN which increases Serca2a activity. These results demonstrate that decreasing phosphorylation of Tpm can rescue the HCM phenotype, presumably by affecting Ca^{2+} cycling mechanisms.

To further examine whether alterations in sarcomeric protein phosphorylation besides Tpm could rescue a HCM phenotype, Alves et al.

[55] crossed the HCM α-Tpm180 mice with pseudo-phosphorylated cardiac TnI mice (TnI-PP). The TnI-PP mice demonstrate a decreased myofilament Ca^{2+} sensitivity compared with wild type myofilaments, whereas, as mentioned previously, the α-Tpm180 HCM mice exhibit an increased Ca^{2+} myofilament sensitivity. When the TnI-PP mice were crossed with the α-Tpm180 mice, the resulting progeny did not develop pathological hypertrophy. Left ventricular performance was improved compared with the α-Tpm180 hearts. Interestingly, there were no changes in Serca2a or PLN expression in the double transgenic mice, but there was increased phosphorylation of PLN and TnT. These results support the hypothesis that reduction in myofilament Ca^{2+} sensitivity through modification of the phosphorylation state of various contractile proteins can delay or prevent the development of HCM.

The previously mentioned studies firmly demonstrate that the pathological cardiac remodeling process can be prevented in the HCM α-Tpm180 mice through a variety of pathways, seemingly all associated with decreasing myofilament Ca^{2+} sensitivity and/or alterations in Ca^{2+} cycling in cardiomyocytes. In a series of experiments designed to test whether the anion exchanger isoform 3 (AE3) could help in the treatment of HCM, we crossed the α-Tpm180 mice with AE3-null mice [56]. Previous work suggested that inhibition of AE3 is protective against cardiac hypertrophy, whereas other studies indicate AE3 is essential for optimal cardiac function. Surprisingly, results show that loss of the AE3 anion exchanger causes increased cardiac remodeling, a more rapid decompensation, and greater severity in heart failure in the double transgenic mice versus the α-Tpm180 transgenic mice alone. This study demonstrates that increased pathological remodeling can occur in the hearts of the α-Tpm180 transgenic mice when subject to additional stresses such as the loss of AE3. Overall, the conclusion drawn from the rescue and advancement of HCM is that cardiac remodeling appears to be a very "plastic" system which is amenable to modification depending upon a number of different factors. Presumably, the direction taken in remodeling is dependent upon various mechanistic changes that occur within the cardiomyocyte to either activate or suppress signaling pathways that modulate stress factors in the heart.

INVOLVEMENT OF TPM IN DILATED CARDIOMYOPATHY REMODELING

Dilated cardiomyopathy (DCM) is a cardiac remodeling process characterized by increased left ventricular volume which often results in stretching and thinning of the ventricular walls; these pathological changes result in decreased systolic function often leading to heart failure. DCM is a relatively common disorder with an incidence of 36.5 out of 100,000 people [57]. Over 50 genetic loci have been identified that are associated with DCM, with these genes encoding nuclear, cytoskeletal and cardiac contractile proteins [58]. With respect to muscle proteins, mutations that lead to DCM have been identified in β-myosin heavy chain, myosin binding protein C, actin, Tpm, TnT, TnI, and TnC, titin, T-cap, desmin, vinculin, and muscle LIM protein [57]. Mutations in α-Tpm were first implicated in causing DCM with the identification of the autosomal dominant missense mutations Glu40Lys and Glu54Lys [59]. Currently, there are at least 12 α-Tpm mutations that are associated with DCM (Figure 1) [31].

In order to better understand the molecular and physiological processes associated with dilated cardiomyopathy remodeling, we generated a transgenic mouse model where we engineered the Glu54Lys mutation in the α-Tpm transgene (α-Tpm54) [60]. A crystal structure of Tpm indicates that Glu54 is linked to Lys49 which is hypothesized to contribute to the stability of the coiled-coil through formation of salt bridges [59]. Disruption of a salt bridge by a DCM mutation could alter the Tpm stability, flexibility, or interactions with actin, thus compromising thin filament integrity or function. Defects in the transmission of force through the thin filament have also been attributed as a cause of DCM [59]. The α-Tpm54 transgenic mouse was the first mouse model in which a mutation in a sarcomeric thin filament protein leads to DCM [60]. Histological and morphological analyses revealed development of DCM with progression to heart failure and frequently death by 6 months. Echocardiographic analyses confirmed the dilated phenotype of the heart with a significant decrease in left ventricular fractional shortening. Work-performing heart analyses showed significantly impaired systolic and diastolic functions, and the force measurements of cardiac myofibers revealed that the myofilament had significantly decreased Ca^{2+} sensitivity and tension generation (Table 1). Reconstituted thin filaments with biochemically exchanged Tpm encoding the DCM mutation also show a decrease in their Ca^{2+} sensitivity [61]. These results confirm the fact that mutations within the same thin filament protein, namely Tpm, can result in cardiac remodeling that is either HCM or DCM dependent upon the specific amino acid substitution that occurs within the protein.

As previously mentioned, α-Tpm is an alternatively spliced gene that generates multiple striated, smooth, and cytoskeletal isoforms. In the human heart, α-Tpm is thought to be the predominant isoform, although the precise composition of Tpm isoform expression was unknown. In an investigation of Tpm expression in human hearts, we confirmed that α-Tpm is the predominant isoform (90–94%), with β-Tpm being expressed at a lower level (3-5%) [14]. Interestingly, we found a unique α-Tpm isoform (α-Tpmκ) is also present in the human heart and expressed at low levels (3-5%) [14]. Surprisingly, additional work found that this α-Tpmκ isoform was increased in patients with DCM and end stage heart failure. These increased levels may serve as a potential non-invasive diagnostic tool in determining the extent of cardiac remodeling that has occurred in a DCM/heart failure patient.

To obtain a better understanding of the morphological and physiological consequences of the α-Tpmκ isoform, we generated transgenic mice to express α-Tpmκ specifically in the heart [14]. Wild type mice do not express endogenous Tpmκ. Results show that increased expression of α-Tpmκ in the heart leads to cardiac remodeling in the form of DCM. Physiological alterations demonstrated a decreased fractional shortening, systolic and diastolic dysfunction, and decreased myofilament Ca^{2+} sensitivity with no change in maximum developed tension (Table 1). Biophysical investigations revealed less structural stability for the α-Tpmκ isoform and weaker actin-binding affinity compared with α-Tpm. These results provide a possible mechanistic explanation for the pathological phenotype that is observed with the Tpm isoform switch that occurs in DCM and heart failure patients.

Tpm Phosphorylation and Cardiac Remodeling

As mentioned previously, Tpm is phosphorylated at a single amino acid, Ser283. To determine whether alterations in phosphorylation status of Tpm would affect myofilament function and cardiac performance, we genetically designed transgenic mice with a Ser283Ala amino acid substitution α-TpmS283A), thereby prohibiting phosphorylation of the exogenous Tpm protein [62, 63]. Results show there was a 86-93% replacement of endogenous Tpm protein with the non-phosphorylatable Tpm. Echocardiographic analysis and cross-sectional area measurements of the α-TpmS283A cardiomyocytes demonstrate a hypertrophic phenotype at basal levels. There are, however, no alterations in cardiac function, myofilament Ca^{2+} sensitivity, cooperativity, or response to β-adrenergic stimulation (Table 1) [62, 63]. Biochemical analyses found there were significant increases in Ca^{2+} handling proteins, specifically in Serca2a and in PLN phosphorylation, which regulate Ca^{2+} sequestration into the SR and sarcomeric contraction. This investigation shows that decreases in Tpm phosphorylation in the heart can result in compensated cardiac hypertrophy.

Recently, we have conducted experiments to determine whether constitutive Tpm phosphorylation may affect sarcomeric performance and cardiac function. These experiments were conducted on transgenic mice which incorporated a phosphor-mimetic (Asp) into the protein (Ser283Asp). Preliminary results show that the hearts from these mice (α-TpmS283D) exhibit a DCM phenotype with diastolic dysfunction, but no alterations in systolic function (Jagatheesan and Wieczorek, unpub results). There were also no changes in Ca^{2+} sensitivity in myofilaments obtained from these transgenic hearts. Collectively, the results from our studies on Tpm phosphorylation in hearts demonstrates that alterations in the sarcomeric Tpm phosphorylation status may have dramatic physiological consequences on cardiac morphology and physiological function that may either be beneficial or pathologic, depending upon the specific circumstances. Additional studies in this area are in progress.

SUMMARY AND CONCLUSION

From the above discussion, it is apparent that various modifications of Tpm can cause extensive cardiac remodeling, mostly associated with HCM or DCM phenotypes. The naturally-occurring Tpm1 (α-Tpm) mutations that are found in human patients are all single amino acid substitutions that lead to sarcomeric dysfunction. These mutations may affect Tpm binding to troponin T or I, or actin; they may also disrupt electrostatic charge interactions between specific amino acids via salt bridges (i.e., Glu54 linkage to Lys49; Glu40 linked to Arg35) [64], disrupting Tpm dimeric interactions and/or binding to troponin and/or actin. These changes may cause a defect in force transmission and result in cardiac remodeling [59]. By altering the biophysical properties of proteins comprising the thin filament, Ca^{2+} binding and release to the myofilament may be disrupted. This is demonstrated most acutely by the alterations in myofilament Ca^{2+} sensitivity that result from α-Tpm mutations. Interestingly, the HCM phenotype has been rescued by various mechanisms that change Ca^{2+} handling and offsetting the effects of the Tpm mutations; these changes have been through increased expression or activity of the Serca2a pump to increase sarcoplasmic reticulum loading of Ca^{2+}. The mechanism by which ablation of Tpm phosphorylation rescues the HCM phenotype is unknown and is currently being investigated. In conclusion, Tpm is an effector of cardiac remodeling – through alterations in Tpm isoforms, mutations, or changes in phosphorylation status, pathological processes are activated which result in the HCM, DCM, or physiological hypertrophy. The precise signaling mechanisms that are activated by these alterations in Tpm and its associated sarcomeric dysfunction is the subject of active inquiry.

REFERENCES

[1] Cohn, J.N., Ferrari, R., and Sharp, N. (2000) Cardiac remodeling – concepts and clinical implications: a consensus paper from an international forum on cardiac remodeling. *J. Am. Coll Cardiol.* 35:569-582.

[2] Spaich, S., Katus H.A., and Backs, J. (2015) Ongoing controversies surrounding cardiac remodeling: is it black and white – or rather fifty shades of gray? *Front. Physiol.* 6:1-15.

[3] Vrhovski, B., Theze, N., and Thiebaud,P. (2008) Structure and evolution of tropomyosin genes. *Adv. Exp. Med. Biol.* 644:6-26.

[4] Hitchcock-DeGregori, S.E. (2008) *Tropomyosin: function follows structure.* In: Gunning, P., editor. Tropomyosin. USA, Springer Science/Landes Bioscience, pp. 60-72.

[5] Muthuchamy, M., Pajak, L., Howles, P., Doetschman, T., and Wieczorek, D.F. (1993) Developmental analysis of tropomyosin gene expression in embryonic stem cells and mouse embryos. *Mol. Cell. Biol.* 13:3311-3323.

[6] Wieczorek, D.F., Smith, C.W., and Nadal-Ginard, B. (1988) The rat α-tropomyosin gene generates a minimum of six different mRNAs coding for striated, smooth, and nonmuscle isoforms by alternative splicing. *Mol. Cell. Biol.* 8:679-694.

[7]   Jagatheesan, G., Rajan, S., and Wieczorek, D.F. (2010) Investigations into tropomyosin function using mouse models. *J. Mol. Cell. Cardiol.* 48:893-898.

[8]   Kee, A.J. and Hardeman, E.C. (2008) Tropomyosin in skeletal muscle diseases. In: Gunning, P., editor. Tropomyosin. USA, Springer Science/Landes Bioscience, pp.143-157.

[9]   Pieples, K. and Wieczorek, D.F. (2000) Tropomyosin 3 increases striated muscle isoform diversity. *Biochem.* 39:8291-8297.

[10]   Wieczorek, D.F., Periasamy M., Butler-Browne, G., Whalen, R., and Nadal-Ginard, B. (1985) Co-expression of multiple myosin heavy chain genes, in addition to a tissue-specific one, in extraocular musculature. *J. Cell Biol.* 101:618-629.

[11]   Moncman, C.L., Andrade, M.E., McCool, A.A., McMullen, C.A., and Andrade, F.H. (2013) Development transitions of thin filament proteins in rat extraocular muscles. *Exp. Cell Res.* 319:23-31.

[12]   Thomas, A., Rajan, S., Thurston H.L., Masineni S.N., Dube, P., Bose, A., Muthu, V., Dube, S., Wieczorek, D.F., and Dube, D.K. (2010) Expression of a novel tropomyosin isoform in axolotl heart and skeletal muscle. *J. Cell Biochem.* 110:875-881.

[13]   Zajdel, R.W., Denz, C.R., Lee, S., Dube, S., Ehler, E., Perriard, E., Perriard, J-C, and Dube, D.K. Identification, characterization, and expression of a novel α-tropomyosin isoform in cardiac tissues in developing chicken. *J. Cell Biochem.* 89:427-439.

[14]   Rajan, S., Jagatheesan, G., Karam, C., Alves, M.L., Bodi, I., Schwartz, A., Bulcao, C., D'Souza, K., Akhter, S., Boivin, G., Dube, D., Petrashevskaya, N., Herr, A., Hullin, R., Liggett, S., Wolska, B., Solaro, R.J., and Wieczorek, D.F. (2010) Molecular and functional characterization of a novel cardiac-specific human tropomyosin isoform. *Circulation* 121:410-418.

[15]   Blanchard, E.M., Iizuka, K., Conner, C., Geisterfer-Lowrance, A., Schoen, F., Maughan, D.W., Seidman, C., and Seidman, J.G. (1997) Targeted ablation of the murine alpha-tropomyosin gene. *Circ. Res.* 81:1005-1010.

[16]   Rethinasamy, P., Muthuchamy, M., Hewett, T., Boivin, G., Wolska, B., Evans, C., Solaro, R.J., and Wieczorek, D.F. (1998) Molecular and physiological effects of α-tropomyosin ablation in the mouse. *Circ. Res.* 82:116-123.

[17]   Hook, J., Lemckert, F., Schevzov, G., Fath, T., and Gunning, P. (2011) Functional identity of gamma tropomyosin gene – implications for

embryonic development, reproduction, and cell viability. *BioArchitecture* 1:49-59.

[18] Muthuchamy, M., Grupp, I., Grupp, G., O'Toole, B., Kier, A., Boivin, G., Neumann, J., and Wieczorek, D.F. (1995) Molecular and physiological effects of overexpressing striated muscle β-tropomyosin in the adult murine heart. *J. Biol. Chem.* 270:30593-30603.

[19] Palmiter, K.A.,Kitada, Y., Muthuchamy, M., Wieczorek, D.F. and Solaro, R.J. (1996) Exchange of β- for α-tropomyosin in hearts of transgenic mice induces changes in thin filament response to Ca^{2+}, strong cross-bridge binding, and protein phosphorylation. *J. Biol. Chem.* 271:11611-11614.

[20] Wolska, B.M., Keller, R.S., Evans, C., Palmiter K., Phillips, R., Muthuchamy, M., Oehlenschlager, J., Wieczorek, D.F., de Tombe, P., and Solaro, R.J. (1999) Correlation between myofilament response to Ca^{2+} and altered dynamics of contraction and relaxation in transgenic cardiac cells that express α-tropomyosin. *Circ. Res.* 84:745-751.

[21] Muthuchamy, M., Boivin, G., Grupp, I., and Wieczorek, D.F. (1998) α-tropomyosin overexpression induces severe cardiac abnormalities. *J. Mol. Cell Cardiol.* 30: 1545-1557.

[22] Jagatheesan, G., Rajan, S., Petrashevskaya, N., Schwartz, A., Bovin, G., Vahebi, S., DeTombe, P., Solaro, R.J., Labitzke, E., Hilliard, G., and Wieczorek, D.F. (2003) Functional importance of the carboxyl-terminal region of striated muscle tropomyosin. *J. Biol. Chem.* 278:23204-23211.

[23] Jagatheesan, G., Rajan, S., Petrashevskaya, N., Schwartz, A., Bovin, G., Arteaga, G., de Tombe, P., Solaro, and Wieczorek, D.F. (2004) Physiological significance of troponin T binding domains in striated muscle tropomyosin. *Am. J. Physiol. Heart Circ. Physiol.* 287:H1484-H1494.

[24] Jagatheesan, G., Rajan, S., Schulz, E., Ahmed, R., Petrashevskaya, N., Schwartz, A., Bovin, G., Arteaga, G., Wang, T., Wang, Y-G., Ashraf, M., Liggett, S., Lorenz, J., Solaro, and Wieczorek, D.F. (2009) An internal domain of α-tropomyosin increases myofilament Ca^{2+} sensitivity. *Am. J. Physiol. Heart Circ. Physiol.* 297:H181-H190.

[25] Pearlstone, J.R., and Smillie, L.B. (1983) Effects of troponin-I plus –C on the binding of troponin-T and its fragments to alpha-tropomyosin Ca^{2+} sensitivity and cooperativity. *J. Biol. Che.* 258:2534-2542.

[26] Zot, A.S. and Potter, J.D. (1987) Structural aspects of troponin-tropomyosin regulation of skeletal muscle contraction. *Annu Rev Biophy Biophy Chem* 16:535-559.

[27] Pieples, K., Arteaga, G., Solaro, R.J., Grupp, I., Lorenz, J., Boivin, G., Jagatheesan, G., Labitzke, E., de Tombe, P., Konhilas, J., Irving, T., and Wieczorek, D.F. (2002) Tropomyosin 3 expression leads to hypercontractility and attenuates myofilament length-dependent Ca^{2+} activation. *Am. J. Physiol Heart Circ. Physiol* 283:H1344-H1353.

[28] Geister-Lowrance, A.A., Kass, S., Tanigawa, G., Vosberg, H.P., McKenna. W., Seidman, D.E., and Seidman, J.G. (1990) A molecular basis for familial hypertrophic cardiomyopathy: a beta cardiac myosin heavy chain gene missense mutation. *Cell* 62:999-1006.

[29] Watkins, H., MacRae, C., Thierfelder, L., Chou, Y.H., Frenneaux, M., McKenna, W., Seidman, J.G., and Seidman, C.E. (1993) A disease locus for familial hypertrophic cardiomyopathy maps to chromosome 1q3. *Nat. Genet.* 3:333-337.

[30] Thierfelder, L., Watkins, H., MacRae, C., Lamas, R., McKenna, W., Vosberg, H.P., Seidman, J.G., and Seidman, C.E. (1994) Alpha-tropomyosin and cardiac troponin T mutations cause familial hypertrophic cardiomyopathy: a disease of the sarcomere. *Cell* 77:701-712.

[31] Redwood, C., and Robinson, P. (2013) Alpha-tropomyosin mutations in inherited cardiomyopathies. *J. Muscle Res. Cell Motil.* 34:285-292.

[32] Tardiff, J.C. Sarcomeric proteins and familial hypertrophic cardiomyopathy: linking mutations in structural proteins to complex cardiovascular phenotypes. *Heart Fail Rev.* 10:237-248.

[33] Nakajima-Taniguichi, C., Matsui, H., Nagata, S., Kishimoto, T., and Yamauchi-Takihara, Y. (1995) Novel missense mutation in α-tropomyosin gene found in Japanese patients with hypertrophic cardiomyopathy. *J. Mol. Cell Cardiol.* 27:2053-2058.

[34] Yamauchi-Takihara, K., Nakajima-Taniguchi, C., Matsui, H., Fujio, R., Kunisada, K., Nagata, S., and Kishimoto, T. (1996) Clinical implications of hypertrophic cardiomyopathy associated mutations in the α-tropomyosin gene. *Heart* 76:63-65.

[35] Jaaskelainen, P., Soranta, M., Miettinen, R., Saarinen, L., Pihlajamaki, J., Silvennoninen, K., Tikanoja, T., Laakso, M., and Kuusisto, J. (1998) The cardiac α-myosin heavy chain gene is not the predominant gene for hypertrophic cardiomyopathy in the Finnish population. *J. Am. Coll Cardiol.* 32:1709-1716.

[36] Bottinelli, R., Coviello, D.A., Redwood, C.S., Pellegrino, M.A., Maron, B.J., Spirito, P., Watkins, H., and Reggiani, C. (1998) A mutant tropomyosin that causes hypertrophic cardiomyopathy is expressed in

vivo and associated with an increased calcium sensitivity. *Circ. Res* 82:106-115.

[37] Muthuchamy, M., Pieples, K., Rethinasamy, P., Hoit, B., Grupp, I., Boivin, G., Wolska, B., Evans, C., Solaro, R.J., and Wieczorek, D.F. (1998) Mouse model of a familial hypertrophic cardiomyopathy mutation in α-tropomyosin manifest cardiac dysfunction. *Circ. Res.* 85:47-56.

[38] Evans, C., Pena, J., Phillips, R., Muthuchamy, M., Wieczorek, D.F., and Solaro, R.J. (2000) Altered hemodynamics in transgenic mice harboring mutant tropomyosin linked to hypertrophic cardiomyopathy. *Am. J. Physiol. Heart Circ. Physiol.* 279:H2414-H2423.

[39] Wermicke, D., Thiel, C., Duja-Isac, C., Essin, K., Spindler, M., Nunez, D., Plehm, R., Wessel, N., Hammes, A., Edwards, R., Lippoldt, A., Zacharias, U., Stromer, H., Neubauer, S., Davies, M., Marano, I., and Thierfelder, L. (2004) Alpha-tropomyosin mutations Asp(175)Asn and Glu(180)Gly affect cardiac function in transgenic rats in different ways. *Am. J. Physiol. Regul Integr. Comp. Physiol.* 287:R685-R695.

[40] Prabhakar, R., Boivin, G., Grupp, I., Hoit, B., Arteaga, G., Solaro, R.J., and Wieczorek, D.F. (2001) A familial hypertrophic cardiomyopathy α-tropomyosin mutation causes severe cardiac hypertrophy and death in mice. *J. Mol. Cell Cardiol.* 33:1815-1828.

[41] Prabhakar, R., Petrashevskaya, N., Schwartz, A., Aronow, B., Boivin, G., Molkentin, J., and Wieczorek, D.F. (2003) A mouse model of familial hypertrophic cardiomyopathy caused by a α-tropomyosin mutation. *Mol. Cell. Biochem.* 251:33-42.

[42] Michele, D., Gomez, C., Hong, K., Westfall, M. and Metzger, J. (2002) Cardiac dysfunction in hypertrophic cardiomyopathy mutant tropomyosin mice is transgene-dependent hypertrophy-independent, and improved by beta-blockade. *Circ. Res.* 91:2550262.

[43] Golitsina, N., An, Y., Greenfield, N., Thierfelder, L., Iizuka, K., Seidman, J., Seidman, C., Lehrer, S., and Hitchcock-DeGregori, S. (1997) Effects of two familial hypertrophic cardiomyopathy-causing mutations on alpha-tropomyosin structure and function. *Biochemistry* 36:4637-4642.

[44] Bing, W., Redwood, C., Purcell, I., Esposito, G., Watkins, H., and Harston, S. (1997) Effects of two hypertrophic cardiomyopathy mutations in alpha-tropomyosin, Asp175Asn and Glu10Gly, on Ca^{2+} regulation of thin filament motility. *Biochem. Biophys. Res. Commun.* 236:760-764.

[45] Bing, W., Knott, A., Redwood C., Esposito, G., Purcell, I., Watkins, H., and Marston, S. (2000) Effect of hypertrophic cardiomyopathy mutations in human cardiac muscle alpha-tropomyosin (Asp175Asn and Glu180Gly) on the regulatory properties of human cardiac troponin determined by in vitro motility assay. *J. Mol. Cell Cardiol.* 32:1489-1498.

[46] Jagatheesan, G., Rajan, S., Petrashevskaya, N., Schwartz, A., Boivin, G., Arteaga, G., Solaro, R.J., Liggett, S., and Wieczorek, D.F. (2007) Rescue of tropomyosin-induced familial hypertrophic cardiomyopathy mice by transgenesis. *Am. J. Physioil. Heart Circ. Physiol.* 293:H949-H958.

[47] Pena, J., Szkudlarek, A., Warren, C., Heinrich, L., Gaffin, R., Jagatheesan, G., del Monte, F., Hajjar, R., Goldspink, P., Solaro, R.J., Wieczorek, D.F., and Wolska, B. (2010) Neonatal gene transfer of Serca2a delays onset of hypertrophic remodeling and improves function in familial hypertrophic cardiomyopathy. *J. Mol. Cell Card.* 49:993-1002.

[48] Byrne, M., Power, J., Preovolos, A., Mariani, J., Hajjar, R., and Kaye, D. (2008) Recirculating cardiac delivery of AAV2/SERCA2a improves myocardial function in an experimental model of heart failure in large animals. *Gene Ther.* 15:1550-1557.

[49] Kawase, Y., Ly, H., Prunier, F., Lebeche, D.,Shi, Y., Jin, H., Hadri, L., Yoneyyama, R., Hoshino, K., Takewa, Y., Sakata, S., Peluso, R., Zsebo, K., Swathmey, J., Tardif, J., Tanguay, J., and Hajjar, R. (2008) Reversal of cardiac dysfunction after long-term expression of SERCA2a by gene transfer in a pre-clinical model of heart failure. *J. Am. Coll. Cardiol.* 51:1112-1119.

[50] Gwathmey, J., Yerevanian, A., and Hajjar, R. (2011) Cardiac gene therapy with SERCA2a: from bench to bedside. *J. Mol. Cell Cardiol* 50:803-812.

[51] Jaski, B., Jessup, M., Mancini, D., Cappola R., Pauly, D., Gfrenberg, B., Borrow, K., Dittrich, H., Zsebo, K., and Hajjar, R. (2009) Calcium upregulation by percutaneous administration of gene therapy in cardiac disease (CUPID trial), a first-in-human phase ½ clinical trial. *J. Card Fail.* 15:171-181.

[52] Gaffin, D., Pena, J., Alves, M., Dias, F., Chowdhury, S., Heinrich, L., Goldspink, P. Kranias, E., Wieczorek, D.F., and Wolska, B.M. (2011) Long-term rescue of a familial hypertrophic cardiomyopathy caused by a

mutation in the thin filament protein, tropomyosin, via modulation of a calcium cycling protein. *J. Mol. Cell Cardiol.* 51:812-820.

[53] Rajan, S., Pena, J., Jegga, A., Aronow B., Wolska, B., and Wieczorek, D.F. (2013) Microarray analysis of active cardiac remodeling genes in a familial hypertrophic cardiomyopathy mouse model rescued by a phospholamban knockout. *Physiol. Genomics* 45:764-773.

[54] Schulz, E., Wilder, T., Chowdhury, S., Sheikh, H., Wolska, B., Solaro, R.J. and Wieczorek, D.F. (2013) Decreasing tropomyosin phosphorylation rescues tropomyosin-induced familial hypertrophic cardiomyopathy. *J. Biol. Chem.* 288:28925-28935.

[55] Alves, M., Dias, F., Gaffin, R., Simon, J., Montminy, E., Biesiadecki, B., Hinken, A., Warren, C., Utter, M., Davis, R., Sakthivel, S., Robbins, J., Wieczorek, D.F., Solaro, R.J., and Wolska, B.M. (2014) Desensitization of myofilaments to Ca^{2+} as a therapeutic target for hypertrophic cardiomyopathy with mutations in thin filament proteins. *Circ. Cardiovasc. Genet.* 7:132-143.

[56] Al Moamen, N., Prasad, V., Bodi, I., Miller, M., Neiman, M., Lasko, V., Alper, S., Wieczorek, D.F., Lorenz, J., and Shull, G. (2011) Loss of the AE3 anion exchanger in a hypertrophic cardiomyopathy model causes rapid decompensation and heart failure. *J. Mol. Cell Cardiol.* 50:137-146.

[57] Chang, A., Harada, K., Ackerman, M., and Potter, J. (2005) Functional consequence of hypertrophic and dilated cardiomyopathy-causing mutations in alpha-tropomyosin. *J. Biol. Chem.* 280:34343-34349.

[58] Watkins, H., Ashrafian, H., and Redwood, C. (2011) Inherited cardiomyopathies. *N. Engl. J. Med.* 364:1643-1656.

[59] Olson, T., Kishimoto, Y., Whitby, F., and Michels, V. (2001) Mutations that alter the surface charge of alpha-tropomyosin are associated with dilated cardiomyopathy. *J. Mol. Cell Cardiol.* 33:723-732.

[60] Rajan, S., Ahmed, R., Jagatheesan G., Petrashevskaya, N., Boivin, G., Urboniene, D., Arteaga, G., Wolska, B., Solaro, R.J. Liggett, and Wieczorek, D.F. (2007) Dilated cardiomyopathy mutant tropomyosin mice develop cardiac dysfunction with significantly decreased fractional shortening and myofilament calcium sensitivity. *Circ. Res.* 101:205-214.

[61] Mirza, M., Robinson, P., Kremneva, E., Copeland, O., Nikolaeva, O., Watkikns, H., Levitsky, D., Redwood, C., El-Mezgueldi, M., and Marston, S. (2007) The effect of mutations in alpha tropomyosin (E40K and E54K), that cause familial dilated cardiomyopathy, on the regulatory

mechanism of cardiac muscle thin filaments. *J. Biol. Chem.* 282:13487-13497.

[62] Schulz, E., Correll, R., Sheikh, H., Lofrano-Alves, M., Engel, P., Newman, G., Schultz, J., Molkentin, J., Wolska, B., Solaro, R.J., and Wieczorek, D.F. (2012) Tropomyosin dephosphorylation results in compensated cardiac hypertrophy. *J. Biol. Chem.* 287:44478-44489.

[63] Schulz, E. and Wieczorek, D.F. (2013) Tropomyosin de-phosphorylation in the heart: what are the consequences? *J. Muscle Res. Cell Motil* 34:239-246.

[64] Brown, J., Kim, K., Jun G., Greenfield, N., Dominguez, R., Wolkmann, N., Hitchcock-DeGregori, S., and Cohen, C. (2001) Deciphering the design of the tropomyosin molecule. *Proc. Natl. Acad. Sci. USA* 98:8496-8501.

In: Cardiac Remodeling
Editor: Jerald Sherman

ISBN: 978-1-63484-270-9
© 2016 Nova Science Publishers, Inc.

Chapter 3

IMPACT OF VITAMIN D SYSTEM ON VENTRICULAR REMODELING

Claudia Kusmic[1], Nicoletta Vesentini[2] and Cristina Barsanti[1]*
[1]Institute of Clinical Physiology, CNR, Pisa, Italy
[2]Abiogen Pharma S.p.A., Pisa, Italy

ABSTRACT

The micronutrient vitamin D has long been appreciated for its role in the homeostasis of bone and in the prevention of rickets. Many studies have shown that vitamin D supplementation may also be effective in the prevention and treatment of disorders of the immune system and inflammation, as well as treatment of diseases such as diabetes, cancer and osteoarthritis. There is growing evidence sustaining an important role for vitamin D on heart health as well.

Recent studies have demonstrated that vitamin D deficiency is very common in patients affected by chronic renal disease or heart failure, and it is associated with poor outcome among these patients. Heart failure has its origins rooted in adverse structural, biochemical and molecular remodeling of myocardium. Vitamin D receptors (VDR) are widespread in the myocardial cellular constituents, including cardiomyocytes, thus justifying an in-depth analysis of how vitamin D accounts for the causes and consequences of adverse heart remodeling. Vitamin D effects are translated at the cellular level through the activation of the specific nuclear receptor by the active

---

* E-mail address: kusmic@ifc.cnr.it.

metabolite of vitamin D, 1,25-dihydroxyvitamin D. Vitamin D is a negative regulator of the renin-angiotensin system and acts to reduce hypertrophic, apoptotic and pro-fibrotic gene expression. Mechanistic insights were gained mainly by experimental studies on VDR-deficient mice, which develop hypertension and adverse cardiac remodeling mediated via the renin-angiotensin system. In addition, studies on mouse models of cardiomyocyte-specific deletion of VDR demonstrated an increase in myocyte size and left ventricular hypertrophy in the conditional knockout.

Given the clinical impact of adverse ventricular remodeling, this review summarizes current knowledge on vitamin D and its biology in heart failure to extend our understanding of factors that may act against ventricular hypertrophy and abnormal geometry.

INTRODUCTION

The name "vitamin D" is applied to a class of different fat-soluble steroid hormones, whose main and well-known functions involve the homeostatic control of calcium and phosphate levels, and the regulation of bone metabolism. As to their chemical structure, they are secosteroids, i.e., steroid molecules with an open ring (Figure 1). In humans, the prevalent active forms are represented by 1,25-dihydroxy-ergocalciferol [$1,25(OH)_2$-vitamin D_2 or $1,25(OH)_2$-D_2], and, above all, by 1,25-dihydroxy-cholecalciferol (also named as calcitriol) [$1,25(OH)_2$-vitamin D_3 or $1,25(OH)_2$-D_3]. As vitamin D_3 can be partly derived from diet and partly produced by endogenous synthesis in the organism under sunlight exposure, the term "vitamin," as referred to an essential nutrient which cannot be synthesized by the body and must be introduced with the diet, is used in this case in an inappropriate way.

The endocrine function of $1,25(OH)_2$-D is essentially associated with the regulation of plasma levels of calcium and phosphate. In particular, given the central role of calcium signaling in a wide variety of cellular, physiological and metabolic processes throughout the whole organism [1], a tight control of calcium balance in the body is of vital importance for health. The maintenance of calcium and phosphate homeostasis is obtained by the interplay of different organ functions, including the bone, the kidney, the intestine and the parathyroid glands, through the actions of different hormonal molecules, as $1,25(OH)_2$-D, parathormone, calcitonin and fibroblast growth factor-23 [2]. The complexity of the network is increased by the fact that each of these hormones interact with the others in feedback circuits in order to exercise a reciprocal modulation on each other's synthesis. Detailed analysis of vitamin

D actions on calcium and phosphate homeostasis can be found in a number of excellent reviews (for example, see: [3, 4]).

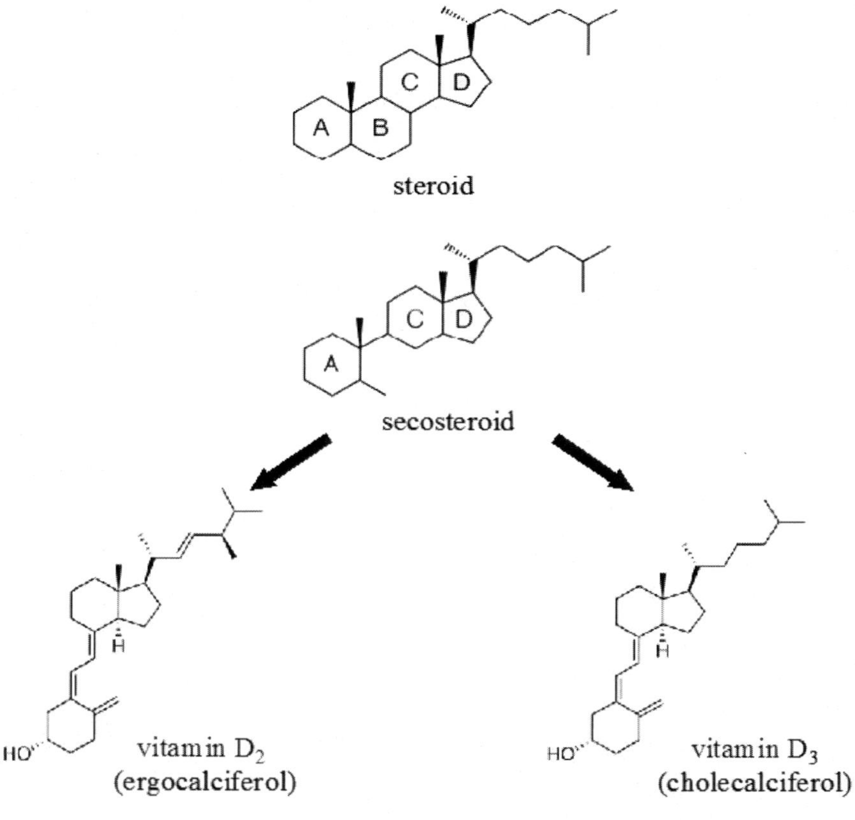

Figure 1. Chemical structure of secosteroids and of the prevalent forms of vitamin D in humans: ergocalciferol (vitamin D_2) and cholecalciferol (vitamin D_3).

Although a severe vitamin D deficiency is associated with defective bone mineralization, provoking rickets in children and osteomalacia in adults, the role of $1,25(OH)_2$-D in bone homeostasis seems to be prevalently indirect, through the control of calcium and phosphate plasmatic levels. This is supported by the fact that these conditions, and similarly bone defects observed in genetic mouse models lacking of the expression of vitamin D receptor (VDR) or of the cytochrome P450 enzyme CYP27B1, responsible for vitamin D conversion to its fully hydroxylated active form, can be rescued by an adequately administration of high calcium and phosphate in the diet [4, 5].

However, many other cells and tissues, apart from those involved in the control of bone and mineral metabolism, have been demonstrated to be capable of directly synthesizing active vitamin D or of responding to vitamin D metabolites. So, in the last decades, research interest about vitamin D has spread far from the original boundaries, as new studies put into light the pleiotropic actions of this hormone in many different contexts associated with human health, such as the regulation of immune system activities, the control of cell proliferation and differentiation, the involvement in the modulation of cardiovascular and metabolic functions [6, 7].

METABOLISM OF VITAMIN D

Diet's contribution as a source of vitamin D generally accounts for a minor part, in the absence of dietary supplements, as adequate amounts of this nutrient are naturally contained in only few foods [8]. Cholecalciferol, which is of animal origin, is found in fatty fish, like salmons and herrings, in eggs, in liver, while lower quantities are present in meat and milk derivatives. Ergocalciferol is mainly contained in mushrooms. Cod liver oil is a particularly relevant source of vitamin D_3 and has been used since the nineteenth century for the prevention of rickets in children, especially in Northern countries with a limited exposure to sunlight during the winter.

The endogenous metabolic pathway of vitamin D_3 involves a series of steps occurring in different body districts, thus requiring the integration of multiple organs' functionality to produce the fully biologically active form of the hormone, $1,25(OH)_2$-cholecalciferol [9, 10] (Figure 2). Light exposure plays a key role in vitamin D synthesis, as the starting point is the photochemical lysis of the precursor 7-dehydrocholesterol to pre-vitamin D_3 by sun radiation in the inner layers of the skin. Specifically, ultraviolet B (UVB) radiation in the wavelength range of 290–315 nm appears to be effective to mediate the reaction. Pre-vitamin D_3 is then rapidly converted by thermal isomerization to cholecalciferol, the inactive form of vitamin D_3. To reach the full biological activity, cholecalciferol must undergo two sequential hydroxylation steps, mainly involving the liver and the kidney.

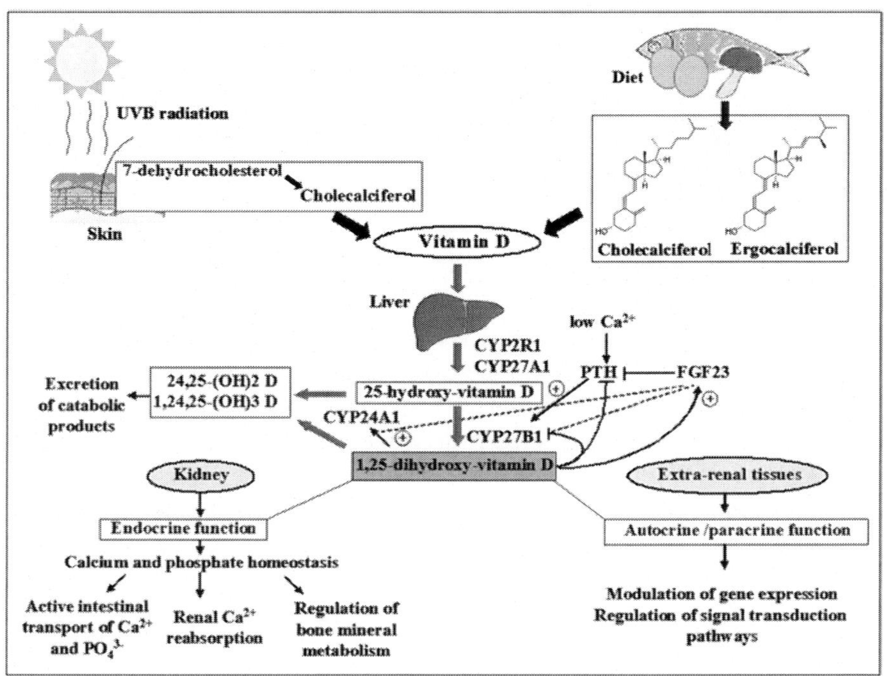

Figure 2. Schematic representation of vitamin D biosynthetic pathway and metabolism. Vitamin D, synthesized in the skin by effect of UVB radiation or introduced with the diet, requires two sequential hydroxylation steps, mediated by cytochrome P450 enzymes, to acquire its full biological activity. The first step occurs in the liver to produce 25(OH)-D, an intermediate with long half-life that is released in the circulation. The fully active hormonal form, 1,25(OH)$_2$-D is produced by action of the CYP27B1 enzyme in the kidney or extra-renal tissues. Renal synthesis is more concerned with the endocrine functions of vitamin D to modulate calcium and phosphate homeostasis in the intestine, kidney and bone. Accordingly, 1,25(OH)$_2$-D production is tightly regulated by a complex interplay with other hormones controlling mineral metabolism, like parathormone (PTH) and fibroblast growth factor-23 (FGF23). In addition, 1,25(OH)$_2$-D levels are known to modulate in reciprocal feedback loops the activity of the biosynthetic CYP27B1 and the catabolic CYP24A1 enzymes. Finally, local production of active vitamin D in a wide variety of tissues is involved in autocrine and paracrine actions, exercised both at genomic and non-genomic level, affecting regulation of gene expression and signal transduction pathways.

Vitamin D, both derived from endogenous synthesis in the skin or from intestinal absorption, enters the blood circulation, where it is prevalently transported through a vitamin D binding protein (DBP). In the liver, cholecalciferol can be converted to 25(OH)-cholecalciferol by several cytochrome P450 hydroxylases, such as CYP2R1 and CYP27A1 [11]. Similarly, ergocalciferol is converted to 25(OH)-ergocalciferol. 25(OH)-vitamin D pro-hormones, as well as the fully hydroxylated active forms, are then released in the circulation and transported by binding with DBP (80-90%) or with albumin (10-20%), while a minor fraction is found as free or unbound [12]. Due to the longer half-life (~3 weeks) and its strict dependence on substrate availability, serum 25(OH)-D measurement is considered to provide the best estimate of a person's vitamin D status respect to the active form. Accordingly, serum 25(OH)-D is usually dosed in the clinic to evaluate deficiency and insufficiency conditions [12].

The conversion of the pro-hormone to the active metabolite $1,25(OH)_2$-D requires a second hydroxylation step that is mediated by the mitochondrial enzyme 25-hydroxyvitamin D-1α-hydroxylase, codified by the *CYP27B1* gene. The proximal tubular epithelial cells in the kidneys represent the main site for production of functional $1,25(OH)_2$-D to be released in the circulation to exercise its broad endocrine activities. However, extra-renal expression of CYP27B1 has also been documented in a wide variety of cells and tissues, such as the monocyte-macrophage system, the placenta, the skin, the brain, and even the cardiac ventricular tissue [13-15].

While $1,25(OH)_2$-D of renal origin is thought to exert a more global action on the bone, intestine and kidney in the maintenance of calcium and phosphate homeostasis, vitamin D synthesized in extra-renal tissues appears to be prevalently involved in autocrine and paracrine functions in the local modulation of gene expression [14].

Finally, the inactivation of vitamin D signaling involves an additional hydroxylation on behalf of the CYP24A1 24-hydroxylase, that is ubiquitously expressed among target tissues. This enzyme mediates the conversion of both 25(OH)-D and $1,25(OH)_2$-D to $24,25(OH)_2$-D and $1,24,25(OH)_3$-D, respectively. Although some biological activity has also been reported for these metabolites in specific contexts, such as in promoting chondrocytes and osteoblasts maturation in culture systems and in processes of bone fracture healing *in vivo* in animal models [16-18], the 24-hydroxylation is primarily considered to represent the first step of the catabolic pathway towards the final conversion into water-soluble and excretable biliary products [11].

VITAMIN D RECEPTOR

Vitamin D receptor (VDR), also known as NR1I1 (nuclear receptor subfamily 1, group I, member 1), is a member of the superfamily of *steroid/thyroid* [19]. 1,25-dihydroxycholecalciferol has a very high affinity for VDR, to which it binds even at subnanomolar concentrations. Upon binding to VDR, $1,25(OH)_2$-D carries out its physiological actions. In mammals, high expression levels of VDR are detected in skin, intestines, kidney, as well as in the thyroid gland [20]. However, sensible expression is found in nearly all tissues, myocardium included [21].

VDR mediates genomic effects of natural or synthetic vitamin D agonists [22]. Indeed, it has been extensively described that upon activation by its ligand, VDR forms heterodimers with the retinoid-X-receptor [23, 24]. The heterodimer thus binds to specific DNA sequences – the vitamin D responsive elements (VDRE) -, usually located in the promoter region of target genes (Figure 3). The prerequisite to direct modulation of transcription by VDR ligands is the location of the activated VDR protein close to the transcription start site (TSS) of the target gene [24]. The heterodimerisation increases DNA-binding efficiency to the VDRE sequence and affects both positive and negative regulation of target genes [25] by inducing local chromatin remodeling, thus promoting or inhibiting the recruitment of the transcriptional machinery to the TSS [19]. Recent research has shown that, in addition to directly controlling the expression of specific target proteins by binding to VDRE motifs on their genomic sequences, VDR regulates also non-coding RNA species, including miRNAs. This could be particularly relevant in order to contemporarily affect the translation of multiple mRNAs into proteins and to coordinate patterns of gene expression, for example, during cell differentiation [26].

The active vitamin D has also been shown to exert fast, non-genomic responses involving stimulation of signal transduction pathways through membrane-associated receptors, which include either the classical VDR receptor, present in association with caveolae in the plasma membrane of some cell types, or a specific membrane-associated rapid response steroid binding receptor ($1,25$-D_3 MARRS) [27-30] (Figure 3). According to the cell type, binding to membrane receptors can induce downstream activation of different intracellular second messengers and signaling pathways, involving protein kinases and phosphatases, phosphoinositide metabolism, G protein-coupled receptors, modulation of ion channels and variations in intracellular calcium levels [9]. Interestingly, even these extra-nuclear signaling pathways contribute, at least to some extent, to the modulation of target gene transcription [9].

In addition, there are evidences that the active form of vitamin D also regulates genes lacking VDR response elements [31] and interacts with other transcription factors such as FoxO and β-catenin [32] as well as exerts post-translational gene regulation by controlling the expression of many proteases and/or protease inhibitors [33].

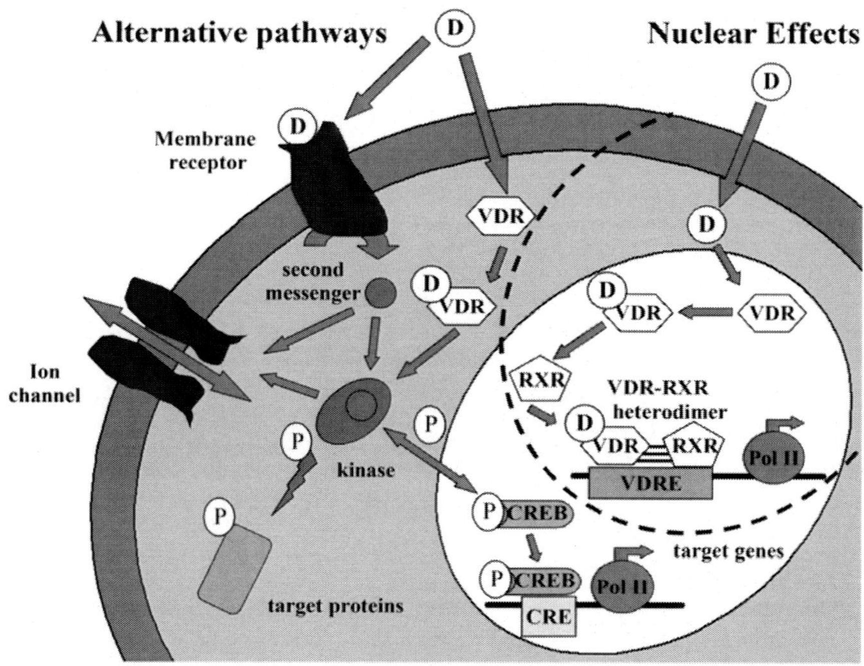

Figure 3. Scheme of the different mechanisms of action of vitamin D. Vitamin D targets appear at 3 different cellular levels. First, there are membrane targets, including receptor(s) related to the membrane-bound vitamin D receptors (VDRs) and non-classic VDRs. The activation of some of these receptors triggers signaling events (e.g., intracellular messengers), resulting in the activation of different kinases. Second, there are cytosolic targets, mainly represented by the classic intracellular VDRs, which activate different signaling pathways. Activation of both membrane and cytosolic targets might ultimately determine a change in gene expression. Finally, there are nuclear targets, defined as the direct modulation of gene expression by the interaction of the VDR-RXR complex with the VDR response element on the DNA. CRE, cAMP response element; CREB, CRE binding protein; VDRE, vitamin D response element; RXR, retinoid X receptor; D, vitamin D; P, phosphate group; Pol II, polymerase II.

VITAMIN D CIRCULATING LEVELS AND CARDIOVASCULAR DISEASE: CLINICAL EVIDENCES

Although there is no general agreement on the optimal circulating level of 25-OH-D, most experts consider a level below 20 ng/ml as a deficiency condition, and levels between 20 and 30 ng/ml as insufficiency. Using this cutoff, the prevalence of insufficiency and deficiency affects respectively 88% and 37% of the population worldwide [34, 35].

In the clinical setting, vitamin D deficiency is a common entity [36, 37] and there are increasing and robust evidences in support of an association between vitamin D deficiency and cardiovascular disease (CVD) [38, 39].

The prevalence of vitamin D deficiency increases with distance from the equator and in a similar manner do the rates of diabetes, hypertension, and CVD. Epidemiologic studies showed a strong association between vitamin D deficiency (and/or reduced VDR activation) and not only CVD risk factors (hypertension, diabetes, metabolic syndrome, left ventricular hypertrophy, atherosclerosis), but also myocardial infarction, and all-cause mortality [40-46]. In addition, vitamin D deficiency, together with secondary hyperparathyroidism, is frequently observed in patients with chronic kidney disease (CKD) and may also contribute to disease progression and cardiovascular disease-related morbidity and mortality [47, 48]. Circulating 25(OH)-D levels are also significantly reduced in patients with heart failure (HF), and are independently associated with poor clinical outcomes [38, 49-52].

Both renin activity and hypertension have been found to be inversely associated with vitamin D levels in clinical observational studies [53-55]. The influence of vitamin D metabolites on renin-angiotensin system suggests an important role in the physiological control of vascular tone and hypertension, and hence in the pathophysiology of cardiac remodeling.

The association between vitamin D and heart function and geometry observed in humans may, however, be an effect by reverse causation, especially in those patients with prevalent heart failure, constrained to a housebound lifestyle and with very limited exposure to sunlight. For this reason, data from prospective studies on the role of vitamin D in subjects without prior heart failure may be distinctive.

Unfortunately, the few studies performed in subjects without known prior myocardial infarctions and/or heart failure are not conclusive in setting a clear relationship between circulating levels of vitamin D and left ventricle (LV) geometry and function, or on the effect of supplementation with vitamin D [53, 56-58]. Moreover, it is commonly known that association does not imply causality. The latter requires consistency of association, biological plausibility, dose-response assays: all conditions that can be tested and verified only through experimental studies.

Further, VDR genetics may also play a role in fibrosis and potentially HF progression. Several polymorphisms in the gene encoding VDR have been identified and associated, together with their allelic combinations, with different degrees of fibrosis in patients with heart failure [59].

VITAMIN D PATHWAY AND CARDIAC HYPERTROPHY

Left ventricular hypertrophy is recognized as one of the strongest risk factors for cardiovascular mortality, and LV remodeling plays a central role in the pathophysiology of advancing heart failure. Although there is growing evidence to suggest an association between vitamin D levels and the development and progression of ventricular remodeling [60], the precise mechanisms explaining such a relationship in HF patients remain unclear.

Mechanistic insights of the effects of vitamin D and its signal transduction system on heart structure and function were gained through several experimental studies over the last decades.

Since the first observation of the beneficial effect of vitamin D supplementation in rats on blood pressure by Briskin et al. [61], many investigations have been performed on experimental models of vitamin D deficiency. Significant changes in myocardial function [62, 63], fibrosis [64], and hypertrophy [63], as well as higher systolic blood pressure [62, 65] were demonstrated in animals fed with vitamin D-deficient diet.

Moreover, genetic studies using mutant mice lacking the vitamin D receptor or the CYP27B1 biosynthetic enzyme have established a correlation between impaired vitamin D system and maladaptive cardiac remodeling, which partly involves the activation of both the systemic and cardiac renin-angiotensin system (RAS), and consequently of angiotensin II [66-69].

Conversely, treatment with vitamin D metabolites attenuated the development of cardiac hypertrophy in hypertensive and uremic rats [70-73] and rescued the cardiac phenotype of *CYP27B1* null mice [68].

A likely mechanism underlying the cardioprotective effects of vitamin D may be the downregulation of RAS. To run through the molecular mechanism, Yuan and coworkers studied the mouse renin gene promoter by luciferase report assay [74]. They found that the active form of vitamin D suppressed the renin gene transcription by blocking the formation of the cyclic AMP/response-element-binding protein complex in the promoter region of the renin gene.

However, the documented expression of VDR on human and animal cardiomyocytes [13, 75] suggests that RAS-independent mechanisms may also contribute to the maladaptive ventricular remodeling, such as myocyte hypertrophy and impaired extracellular matrix homeostasis. To differentiate the secondary effect of hypertension from the direct effect of vitamin D system on ventricular hypertrophy, Chen and coworkers have recently developed a mouse with selective cardiomyocyte deletion of VDR and were able to confirm a direct *in vivo* antihypertrophic action of $1,25(OH)_2$-D [69]. The activation of VDR has been demonstrated to attenuate cardiac fibrosis by lowering the expression of pro-fibrotic genes and to protect from diastolic dysfunction in a murine model of ventricular pressure overload leading to remodeling and heart failure [76]. Moreover, studies using the VDR knock-out mouse model indicated that vitamin D pathway downregulates the cardiac expression of matrix metalloproteinases (MMPs) and the associated collagen deposition and fibrosis in the cardiac tissue [77]. In addition, $1,25(OH)_2$-D_3 inhibits the TGFβ1-mediated activation of primary ventricular human cardiac fibroblasts [78]. Vitamin D pathway has also been demonstrated to inhibit the expression of hypertrophy-sensitive genes, such as those encoding the atrial natriuretic peptide (ANP) in neonatal atrial and ventricular myocyte cells [79-81]. The mechanism of inhibition is likely provided by a protein-protein interaction between the liganded VDR and positive transcription factors of the ANP gene rather than a direct interaction between the activated VDR and the regulatory elements in the gene promoter region [82].

Whole heart and cellular preparations from animal models have been studied to better understand the influence of vitamin D on contractile function and intracellular calcium levels. Increased contraction and relaxation rates – which in live intact animals would appear as changes in cardiac heart rate parameters associated with the compensatory phase of the failing heart - were paradoxically measured in isolated perfused hearts from rats fed with vitamin D-depleted diet [62] and in cardiomyocytes isolated from VDR-knockout mice [83]. In adult rodent cardiomyocytes, VDR is located in the t-tubular structure of sarcolemma. Upon activation by calcitriol, a portion of the receptor translocates to the nucleus to modulate genomic effects. However, the interaction of membrane-bound VDR and caveolin-3 in the t-tubules may also explain the fast, non-genomic mechanism to control myocyte contractile function through the regulation of cellular Ca^{2+} cycling [84]. The acute effect of calcitriol is mainly to accelerate relaxation [83, 85], which suggests that the integrity of vitamin D system is important for the preservation of diastolic function.

VDR deficiency results in the chronic impairment of contractile kinetics and the absence of rapid effects on sarcomere contraction upon vitamin D treatment [83]. There are several mechanism by which vitamin D and VDR pathway may affect myocyte Ca^{2+} handling. $1,25(OH)_2$-D_3 directly stimulates calcium influx through Ca^{2+} channels in cultured chick and rat cardiac cells [86, 87]. Cellular Ca^{2+} currents and Ca^{2+} handling regulatory proteins may also be modulated by the non-genomic action of calcitriol through protein kinase A and C and β_2-adrenergic signaling pathways [85, 88-90]. However, the fast effect of vitamin D on myocyte contraction is blocked only by inhibition of PKC indicating a leading role of PKC signaling in this process [85].

Vitamin D is also considered an important hormone involved in modulation and upkeep of myocyte structure and function as well as in cardiac tissue growth and development. Vitamin D reduces proliferation without promoting apoptosis, downregulates the expression of *c-myc* and genes related to the cell cycle (cyclins A1, C, and E and cyclin-dependent kinases Cdk2 and Cdk4) in cardiac cells in culture [91-94]. However, as the results have been obtained in cultured cells and, in some cases in neonatal or immortalized myocyte cell lines, whereas cardiomyocytes in the cardiac tissue rarely divide, it is unclear whether the same effects would be observed *in vivo*.

CONCLUSION

It is now clear that vitamin D plays a pivotal role in cardiovascular health via traditional and non-traditional CVD risk factors. Several studies suggest that vitamin D exerts important effects on cardiac tissue through regulation of cell contraction, intracellular calcium handling, myocyte proliferation and ECM homeostasis. All these important effects are mediated by both non-genomic and genomic signaling pathways associated to VDR expressed on cardiomyocytes. Although the great majority of data have been obtained in animal models or cell cultures and the direct translation of the results to the human situation needs to be confirmed, the vitamin D receptor has also been identified in human heart tissue [95]. Hence, it is likely that many of the mechanistic molecular pathways may be common and thus making the effects of vitamin D on cardiac function observed in rodents also relevant to humans.

A better understanding of the molecular signaling through which vitamin D impacts on ventricular remodeling in humans may provide useful advances for the development of targeted therapies and prospective clinical interventions.

REFERENCES

[1] M. J. Berridge, M. D. Bootman and H. L. Roderick. *Nat. Rev. Mol. Cell Biol.* 4, 517 (2003).

[2] R. Civitelli and K. Ziambaras. *J. Endocrinol. Invest.* 34, 3 (2011).

[3] L. Lieben, G. Carmeliet and R. Masuyama. *Best Pract. Res. Clin. Endocrinol. Metab.* 25, 561 (2011).

[4] P. H. Anderson, A. G. Turner and H. A. Morris. *Clin. Biochem.* 45, 880 (2012).

[5] R Bouillon, G. Carmeliet, L. Verlinden, E. van Etten, A. Verstuyf, H. F. Luderer, L. Lieben, C. Mathieu and M. Demay. *Endocr. Rev.* 29, 726 (2008).

[6] A. Verstuyf, G. Carmeliet, R. Bouillon and C. Mathieu. *Kidney Int.* 78, 140 (2010).

[7] Y. H. Lai and T. C. Fang. *ISRN Nephrol.* 2013/898125, eCollection (2013).

[8] I. Bendik, A. Friedel, F. F. Roos, P. Weber and M. Eggersdorfer. *Front. Physiol.* 5, 248 (2014).

[9] A. W. Norman. *Am. J. Clin. Nutr.* 88, 491S (2008).

[10] J. S. Adams, J. Ramin, B. Rafison, C. Windon, A. Windon and P. T. Liu. *Bone Res.* 1, 2 (2013).

[11] G. Jones, D. E. Prosser and M. Kaufmann. *J. Lipid Res.* 55, 13 (2014).

[12] J. E. Zerwekh. *Am. J. Clin. Nutr.* 87, 1087S (2008).

[13] S. Chen, D. J. Glenn, L. W. Ni, C. L. Grigbsby, K. Olsen, M. Nishimoto, C. S. Law and D. G. Gardner. *Hypertension* 52, 1106 (2008).

[14] H. A. Morris and P. H. Anderson. *Clin. Biochem. Rev.* 31, 129 (2010).

[15] J. S. Adams and M. Hewison. *Arch. Biochem. Biophys.* 523, 95 (2012).

[16] B. D. Boyan, V. L. Sylvia, D. D. Dean, and Z. Schwartz. *Steroids* 66, 363 (2001).

[17] R. St-Arnaud. *J. Steroid Biochem. Mol. Biol.* 121, 254 (2010).

[18] K. M. Curtis, K. K. Aenlle, B. A. Roos and G. A. Howard. *Mol. Endocrinol.* 28, 644 (2014).

[19] C. Carlberg and M. J. Campbell. *Steroids* 78, 127 (2013).

[20]   A. L. Bookout, Y. Jeong, M. Downes, R. T. Yu, R. M. Evans and D. J. Mangelsdorf. *Cell* 126, 789 (2006).

[21]   T. Yao, X. Ying, Y. Zhao, A. Yuan, Q. He, H. Tong, S. Ding, J. Liu, X. Peng, E. Gao, J. Pu and B. He. *Antioxid. Redox Signal.* 22, 633 (2015).

[22]   A. Franczyk, K. Stolarz-Skrzypek, A. Wesołowska and D. Czarnecka. *Cardiovasc. Hematol. Disord. Drug Targets* 14, 34 (2014).

[23]   M. Schräder, I. Bendik, M. Becker-André and C. Carlberg. *J. Biol. Chem.* 268, 17830 (1993).

[24]   C. Carlberg and S. Seuter. *Anticancer Res.* 29, 3485 (2009).

[25]   A. Hossein-nhezad, A. Spira and M. F. Holick. *PLoS One* 8, e58725 (2013).

[26]   M. D. Long, L. E. Sucheston-Campbell and M. J. Campbell. *J. Cell Physiol.* 230, 758 (2015).

[27]   A. De Boland and R. Boland. *Biochim. Biophys. Acta* 1179, 98 (1993).

[28]   A. De Boland, S. Morelli and R. Boland. *J. Biol. Chem.* 269, 8675 (1994).

[29]   D. Capiati, S. Benassati and R. L. Boland. *J. Cell Biochem.* 86, 128 (2002).

[30]   R. C. Khanal and I. Nemere. *Crit. Rev. Eukaryot. Gene Expr.* 17, 31 (2007).

[31]   R. St-Arnaud, G. A. Candeliere and S. Dedhar. *Front. Biosci.* 1, d177 (1996).

[32]   M. DeWitt, R. L. Johnson, P. Snyder and J. C. Fleet. *J. Steroid Biochem. Mol. Biol.* 148, 103 (2015).

[33]   M. R. Haussler, P. W. Jurutka, M. Mizwicki and A. W. Norman. *Best Pract. Res. Clin. Endocrinol. Metab.* 25, 543 (2011).

[34]   M. F. Holick, N. C. Binkley, H. A. Bischoff-Ferrari, C. M. Gordon, D. A. Hanley, R. P. Heaney, M. H. Murad and C. M. Weaver. *J. Clin. Endocrinol. Metab.* 96, 1911 (2011).

[35]   J. Hilger, A. Friedel, R. Herr, T. Rausch, F. Roos, D. A. Wahl, D. D. Pierroz, P. Weber and K. Hoffmann. *Br. J. Nutr.* 111, 23 (2014).

[36]   E. Kristal-Boneh, P. Froom, G. Harara and J. Ribak. *Hypertension* 30, 1289 (1997).

[37]   M. F. Holick. *Mol. Aspects Med.* 29, 361 (2008).

[38]   A. Zittermann, S. S. Schleithoff, G. Tenderich, H. K. Berthold, R. Korfer, P. Stehle. *J. Am. Coll. Cardiol.* 41, 105 (2003).

[39]   A. Zittermann, S. S. Schleithoff, C. Gotting, O. Dronow, U. Fuchs, J. Kuhn, K. Kleesiek, G. Tenderich and R. Koerfer. *Eur. J. Heart Fail.* 10, 321 (2008).

[40] R. Scragg, R. Jackson, I. M. Holdaway, T. Lim and R. Beaglehole. *Int. J. Epidemiol.* 19, 559 (1990).

[41] A. C. Looker, B. Dawson-Hughes, M. S. Calvo, E. W. Gunter and N. R. Sahyoun. *Bone* 30, 77 (2002).

[42] M. F. Holick. *N. Engl. J. Med.* 357, 266 (2007).

[43] D. Martins, M. Wolf, D. Pan, A. Zadshir, N. Tareen, R. Thadhani, A. Felsenfeld, B. Levine, R. Mehrotra and K. Norris. *Arch. Intern. Med.* 167, 1159 (2007).

[44] H. Dobnig, S. Pilz, H. Scharnagl, W. Renner, U. Seelhorst, B. Wellnitz, J. Kinkeldei, B. O. Boehm, G Weihrauch and W. Maerz. *Arch. Intern. Med.* 168, 1340 (2008).

[45] E. Giovannucci, Y. Liu, B. W. Hollis and E. B. Rimm. *Arch. Intern. Med.* 168, 1174 (2008).

[46] J. Oh, S. Weng, S. K. Felton, S. Bhandare, A. Riek, B. Butler, B. M. Proctor, M. Petty, Z. Chen, K. B. Schechtman, L. Bernal-Mizrachi and C. Bernal-Mizrachi. *Circulation* 120, 687 (2009).

[47] A. S. Go, G. M. Chertow, D. Fan, C. E. McCulloch and C. Hsu. *N. Engl. J. Med.* 351, 1296 (2004).

[48] A. Verma, N. S. Anavekar, A. Meris, J. J. Thune, J. M. Arnold, J. K. Ghali, E. J. Velazquez, J. J. McMurray, M. A. Pfeffer and S. D. Solomon. *J. Am. Coll. Cardiol.* 50, 1238 (2007).

[49] L. C. Liu, A. A. Voors, D. J. van Veldhuisen, E. van der Veer, A. M. Belonje, M. K. Szymanski, H. H. Sillje, W. H. van Gilst, T. Jaarsma and R. A. de Boer. *Eur. J. Heart Fail.* 13, 619 (2011).

[50] L. L. Schierbeck, T. S. Jensen, U. Bang, G. Jensen, L. Kober and J. E. Jensen. *Eur. J. Heart Fail.* 13, 626 (2011).

[51] I. Gotsman, A. Shauer, D. R. Zwas, Y. Hellman, A. Keren, C. Lotan and D. Admon. *Eur. J. Heart Fail.* 14, 357 (2012).

[52] D. Gruson, B. Ferracin, S. A. Ahn, C. Zierold, F. Blocki, D. M. Hawkins, F. Bonelli and M. F. Rousseau. *PLoS One.* 10, e0135427 (2015).

[53] S. Pilz, R. M. Henry, M. B. Snijder, R. M. van Dam, G. Nijpels, C. D. Stehouwer, O. Kamp, A. Tomaschitz, T. R. Pieber and J. M. Dekker. *J. Endocrinol. Invest.* 33, 612 (2010).

[54] A. Burgaz, N. Orsini, S. C. Larsson and A. Wolk. *J. Hypertens.* 29, 636 (2011).

[55] A. Vaidya, J. P. Forman, P. N. Hopkins, E. W. Seely, J. S. Williams. *J. Renin Angiotensin Aldosterone Syst.* 12, 311 (2011).

[56] T. Fall, I. Shiue, P. Bergeå af Geijerstam, J. Sundström, J. Ärnlöv, A. Larsson, H. Melhus, L. Lind and E. Ingelsson. *Eur. J. Heart Fail.* 14, 985 (2012).

[57] A. J. van Ballegooijen, M. B. Snijder, M. Visser, K. van den Hurk, O. Kamp, J. M. Dekker, G. Nijpels, C. D. Stehouwer, R. M. Henry, W. J. Paulus and I. A. Brouwer. *Ann. Nutr. Metab.* 60, 69 (2012).

[58] U. Canpolat, F. Özcan, Ö. Özeke, O. Turak, Ç. Yayla, S. K. Açıkgöz, S. Çay, S. Topaloğlu, D. Aras and S. Aydoğdu. *Ann. Noninvasive Electrocardiol.* 20, 378 (2015).

[59] M. P. Dorsh, C. W. Nemerovski, V. L. Ellingrod, J. A. Cowger, D. B. Dyke, T. M. Koelling, A. H. Wu, K. D. Aaronson, R. U. Simpson and B. E. Bleske. *J. Cardiovasc. Pharmacol. Ther.* 19, 439 (2014).

[60] L. M. Meems, P. van der Harst, W. H. van Gilst and R. A. de Boer. *Curr. Drug Targets* 12, 29 (2011).

[61] H.L. Briskin, F.R. Stokes, C.I. Reed and R.G. Mrazek. *Am. J. Physiol.* 138, 385 (1943).

[62] R. E. Weishaar and R. U. Simpson. *J. Clin. Invest.* 79, 1706 (1987).

[63] H. B. Assalin, B. P. Rafacho, P. P. dos Santos, L. P. Ardisson, M. G. Roscani, F. Chiuso-Minicucci, L. F. Barbisan, A. A. Fernandes, P. S. Azevedo, M. F. Minicucci, L. A. Zornoff and S. A. de Paiva. *Circ. Heart Fail.* 6, 809 (2013).

[64] R. E. Weishaar, S. N. Kim, D. E. Saunders and R. U. Simpson. *Am. J. Physiol.* 258, E134 (1990).

[65] F. Sundersingh, L. A. Plum and H. F. DeLuca. *Biochem. Biophys. Res. Commun.* 461, 589 (2015).

[66] Y. C. Li, J. Kong, M. Wei, Z. F. Chen, S. Q. Liu and L. P. Cao. *J. Clin. Invest.* 110, 229 (2002).

[67] W. Xiang, J. Kong, S. Chen, L. P. Cao, G. Qiao, W. Zheng, W. Liu, X. Li, D. G. Gardner and Y. C. Li. *Am. J. Physio.l Endocrinol. Metab.* 288, E125 (2005).

[68] C. Zhou, F. Lu, K. Cao, D. Xu, D. Goltzman and D. Miao. *Kidney Int.* 74, 170 (2008).

[69] S. Chen, C. S. Law, C. L. Grigsby, K. Olsen, T. T. Hong, Y. Zhang, Y. Yeghiazarians and D. G. Gardner. *Circulation* 124, 1838 (2011).

[70] N. Bodyak, J. C. Ayus, S. Achinger, V. Shivalingappa, Q. Ke, Y. S. Chen, D. L. Rigor, I. Stillman, H. Tamez, P. E. Kroeger, R. R. Wu-Wong, S. A. Karumanchi, R. Thadhani and P. M. Kang. *Proc. Natl. Acad. Sc.i USA* 104, 16810 (2007).

[71] J. Kong, G. H. Kim, M. Wei, T. Sun, G. Li, S. Q. Liu, X. Li, I. Bhan, Q. Zhao, R. Thadhani and Y. C. Li. *Am. J. Pathol.* 177, 622 (2010).

[72] S. Bae, B. Yalamarti, Q. Ke, S. Choudhury, H. Yu, S. A. Karumanchi, P. Kroeger, R. Thadhani and P. M. Kang. *Cardiovasc. Res.* 91, 632 (2011).

[73] M. Freundlich, Y. C. Li, Y. Quiroz, Y. Bravo, W. Seeherunvong, C. Faul, J. R. Weisinger and B. Rodriguez-Iturbe. *Am. J. Hypertens.* 27, 720 (2014).

[74] W. Yuan, W. Pan, J. Kong, W. Zheng, F. L. Szeto, K. E. Wong, R. Cohen, A. Klopot, Z. Zhang and Y. C. Li. *J. Biol. Chem.* 282, 29821 (2007).

[75] R. U. Simpson, G. A. Thomas and A. J. Arnold. *J. Biol. Chem.* 260, 8882 (1985).

[76] L. M. Meems, M. V. Cannon, H. Mahmud, A. A. Voors, W. H. van Gilst, H. H. Silljé, W. P. Ruifrok and R. A. de Boer. *J. Steroid Biochem. Mol. Biol.* 132, 282 (2012).

[77] A. Rahman, S. Hershey, S. Ahmed, K. Nibbelink and R. U. Simpson. *J. Steroid Biochem. Mol. Biol.* 103, 416 (2007).

[78] A. Meredith, S. Boroomand, J. Carthy, Z. Luo and B. McManus. *PLoS One* 10, e0128655 (2015).

[79] Q. Li and D. G. Gardner. *J. Biol. Chem.* 269, 4934 (1994).

[80] J. Wu, M. Garami, L. Cao, Q. Li and D. G. Gardner. *Am. J. Physiol.* 268, 1108 (1995).

[81] J. Wu, M. Garami, T. Cheng and D. G. Gardner. *J. Clin. Invest.* 97, 1577 (1996).

[82] S. Chen, K. Nakamura and D. G. Gardner. *Regul. Pept.* 128, 197 (2005).

[83] D. X. Tishkoff, K. A. Nibbelink, K. H. Holmberg, L. Dandu and R. U. Simpson. *Endocrinology.* 149, 558 (2008).

[84] G. Zhao and R. U. Simpson. *J. Steroid Biochem. Mol. Biol.* 121, 159 (2010).

[85] J. J. Green, D. A. Robinson, G. E. Wilson, R. U. Simpson and M. V. Westfall. *J. Mol. Cell Cardiol.* 41, 350 (2006).

[86] M. R. Walters, T.T. Ilenchuk and W. C. Claycomb. *J. Biol. Chem.* 262, 2536 (1987).

[87] J. Sellés, T. Bellido and R. L. Boland. *J. Mol. Cell Cardiol.* 26, 1593 (1994).

[88] J. Sellés and R. L. Boland. *Mol. Cell Endocrinol.* 82, 229 (1991).

[89] G. E. Santillan and R. L. Boland. *J. Mol. Cell Cardiol.* 30, 225 (1998).

[90] G. E. Santillan, G. Vazquez and R. L. Boland. *J. Mol. Cell Cardiol.* 31, 1095 (1999).

[91] T. D. O'Connell, J. E. Berry, A. K. Jarvis, M. J. Somerman and R. U. Simpson. *Am. J. Physiol.* 272, H1751 (1997).

[92] K. A. Nibbelink, D. X, Tishkoff, S. D. Hershey, A. Rahman and R. U. Simpson. *J. Steroid Biochem. Mol. Biol.* 103, 533 (2007).

[93] J. N. Artaza and K. C. Norris *J. Investig. Med.* 57, 112 (2009).

[94] S. M. Hlaing, L. A. Garcia, J. R. Contreras, K. C. Norris, M. G. Ferrini and J. N. Artaza. *J. Mol. Endocrinol.* 53, 303 (2014).

[95] T. D. O'Connell and R. U. Simpson. *Cell Biol. Int.* 20, 621 (1996).

In: Cardiac Remodeling
Editor: Jerald Sherman

ISBN: 978-1-63484-270-9
© 2016 Nova Science Publishers, Inc.

Chapter 4

EFFECTS OF COFFEE POLYPHENOLS ON MYOCARDIAL REMODELING

Jun-ichi Suzuki[*]
Department of Advanced Clinical Science and Therapeutics,
The University of Tokyo, Tokyo, Japan

ABSTRACT

It is well known that moderate coffee intake inhibits the development of cardiovascular diseases in clinical settings. However, the effect of chlorogenic acid (CGA), one of the major polyphenol constituents of coffee beans, on the disease is yet to be elucidated. This article reviews the effect of CGA on myocardial remodeling. Firstly, we reviewed the effects of CGA on human cardiovascular diseases. Several studies indicated that CGA might decrease the clinical risk of cardiovascular diseases via anti-hypertensive and anti-endothelial dysfunction. Next, we demonstrated that CGA could improve pathological remodeling through the suppression of myocardial cell infiltration and fibrosis in animal models. Our findings and previous data suggest that the CGA treatment may have beneficial effects on the progression of myocardial remodeling.

Keywords: coffee extract, polyphenol, heart, inflammation, remodeling

---

[*] Correspondence to Jun-ichi Suzuki: 7-3-1 Hongo, Bunkyo, Tokyo 113-8655, Japan; Phone, 81-3-5800-9116; Fax, 81-3-5800-9182; e-mail, junichisuzuki-circ@umin.ac.jp.

1. Introduction

A major polyphenol constituent of coffee beans, chlorogenic acid (CGA) is a potent anti-oxidant and anti-inflammatory substance [1, 2]. These effects are induced by the suppression of inflammatory factors, including nuclear factor-kappa B (NF-κB) [3, 4]. Resent data has also indicated that CGA inhibits interleukin (IL)-1β and tumor necrosis factor (TNF)-α production in animals with rheumatoid arthritis [5]. However, the effect of CGA on myocardial remodeling is yet to be elucidated. Therefore, this article reviews the effect of CGA on myocardial remodeling.

2. Effects of CGA on Cardiovascular Diseases in Clinical Studies

European studies showed that moderate coffee drinking reduced cardiovascular risk by 31% relative to no consumption. However, over consumption of coffee significantly increased the risk [6]. A similar J-curve was also observed in a Finnish study [7]. A study of over 40,000 post-menopausal US women showed the hazard ratio of death attributed to cardiovascular diseases was 0.76 for consumption of 1–3 cups/day, 0.81 for 4–5 cups/day, and 0.87 for ≥6 cups/day [8]. Thus, moderate consumption of coffee may inhibit inflammation and reduce the risk of cardiovascular and other inflammatory diseases.

Few clinical studies of CGA's influence on cardiovascular diseases have been performed. A study showed that the CGA significantly lowered systolic and diastolic blood pressure compared with the placebo group [9]. Normotensive subjects with reduced vasoreactivity were also administered with CGA. There was a significant decrease in plasma homocysteine compared with the baseline value for the CGA group [10]. These results indicate that CGA may decrease the risk of cardiovascular diseases.

3. Effects of CGA on Cardiovascular Diseases in Animal Studies

A study showed the effect of CGA on spontaneously hypertensive rats. A single ingestion of CGA reduced blood pressure in the rats, an effect that was blocked by administration of a nitric oxide synthase inhibitor. When spontaneously hypertensive rats were fed diets containing 0.5% CGA for 8 weeks, the development of hypertension was inhibited compared with the control diet group. Dietary CGA also reduced oxidative stress and improved nitric oxide bioavailability by inhibiting excessive production of reactive oxygen species in the vasculature, and led to the attenuation of endothelial dysfunction [11]. At a more relevant dose, CGA given to mice at 10 mg/kg activated calcineurin and enhanced macrophage functions in normal mice, a possible cardiac benefit [12].

4. CGA ON MYOCARDIAL INFARCTION

The mortality rate in patients with coronary arterial disease, including myocardial infarction (MI), is high [13]. Myocardial necrosis and ventricular remodeling after MI lead to arrhythmia, cardiac rupture and heart failure. Many studies showed that macrophage related inflammatory response increased myocardial necrosis [14, 15]. These inflammatory responses lead to an increase of fibroblasts and collagen synthesis [16-19]. To test the hypothesis that CGA can attenuate chronic ventricular remodeling after myocardial ischemia, we performed oral administration of CGA into murine myocardial ischemia models. The MI model was produced by permanent ligation of the left anterior descending coronary artery. Some MI mice were supplemented orally with CGA as a CGA-treated MI group, and other MI mice received vehicle as a vehicle-treated MI group. Sham-operated mice without MI also received vehicle as a sham group, and sham-operated mice without MI received CGA as a Sham + CGA group. Just before sacrifice on day 14, we measured blood pressure, heart rate, and echocardiogram. We revealed the vehicle-treated MI group showed significantly impaired left ventricular contraction compared to the sham-operated group. However, the CGA-treated MI group showed significantly improved ventricular contraction compared to the vehicle-treated MI group. Severe myocardial fibrosis with enhanced macrophage infiltration was observed in the vehicle-treated ischemia group. CGA attenuated these fibrotic changes with suppressed macrophage infiltration without systemic adverse effects. We concluded that CGA might effectively suppress chronic ventricular remodeling after myocardial ischemia because it is critically involved in the suppression of macrophage infiltration [20].

5. CGA ON MYOCARDITIS

Myocarditis is another serious myocardial disease. Patients with myocarditis in its severest form may suffer from rapidly progressive heart failure, shock, arrhythmia, or death [21-26]. In patients with myocarditis, autoimmune disease is considered to be responsible for the pathogenesis [27-29]. Autoimmune myocarditis can be induced in mice or rats by immunization with cardiac myosin [27, 28, 30]. This model revealed that reactive oxygen species and inflammation are key modulators of myocarditis [28, 31, 32].

A cell adhesion glycoprotein molecule, intercellular adhesion molecule (ICAM)-1 revealed upregulation of ligand expression by inflammatory cytokines as an important switch to initiate adhesion [33]. It has shown that ICAM-1 associates pathological process of myocarditis [34, 35]. It was reported that ICAM-1 in myocardial cells plays a critical role in the acute viral myocarditis that investigated using ICAM-1 neutralizing antibody [34]. Resent data also revealed that ICAM-1 is expressed by inflammation and ROS [36, 37]. Therefore, it suggests that ICAM-1 is required for the onset of myocarditis. To investigate the effect of CGA on myocarditis, we used a murine model of experimental autoimmune myocarditis (EAM). Balb/c mice were immunized with cardiac myosin peptides and complete Freund's adjuvant. CGA or vehicle was administered orally from day 0 to day 21 and the animals were sacrificed on day 21. We demonstrated that CGA significantly suppressed ICAM-1 expression in the EAM hearts. The suppressed ICAM-1 tended to reduce myocardial fibrosis compared to control EAM hearts. The findings suggest CGA influences inhibition of cell adhesion in myocarditis, and may have beneficial effects on the progression of myocarditis [38].

6. FUTURE PERSPECTIVES

Previous investigations have clarified that transcription factors and adhesion molecules are key members in the pathophysiology of myocardial diseases. We have demonstrated that CGA intake significantly suppresses the expression of inflammatory factors including adhesion molecules. These key factors are known to be regulated by NF-κB, which is a central mediator for the development of inflammatory diseases. We have reported specific inhibition of NF-κB using a decoy oligonucleotide had significant therapeutic effects in the myocardial ischemia [39], myocarditis [40], and heart transplant rejection [41]. In these studies, the NF-κB decoy suppresses many inflammatory factors including adhesion molecules. Although CGA is not a specific inhibitor of NF-κB, they have similar effects to the inhibitors such as suppression of adhesion molecules and other inflammatory factors. Therefore, CGA has the potential to treat and/or prevent clinical inflammatory diseases.

CONCLUSION

Our findings and previous data suggest that the CGA treatment may have beneficial effects on the progression of myocardial remodeling.

ACKNOWLEDGMENTS

We would like to thank Ms. Noriko Tamura and Ms. Yasuko Matsuda for their excellent technical assistance.

Grants

This study was supported by the grants from Nestle Nutrition Council Foundation, Ryoshoku, the Food Science Institute Foundation, and the Foundation for Dietary Scientific Research, and All Japan Coffee Association.

REFERENCES

[1]   Bouayed, J.; Rammal, H.; Dicko, A.; Younos, C.; Soulimani, R. Chlorogenic acid, a polyphenol from Prunus domestica (Mirabelle), with coupled anxiolytic and antioxidant effects. *J. Neurol. Sci.* 2007, 262, 77-84.

[2]   Granado-Serrano, A.B.; Martin, M.A.; Izquierdo-Pulido, M.; Goya, L.; Bravo, L.; Ramos, S. Molecular mechanisms of (-)-epicatechin and chlorogenic acid on the regulation of the apoptotic and

survival/proliferation pathways in a human hepatoma cell line. *J. Agric. Food. Chem.* 2007, 55, 2020-7.

[3]   Feng, R.; Lu, Y.; Bowman, L.L.; Qian, Y.; Castranova, V.; Ding, M. Inhibition of activator protein-1, NF-kappaB, and MAPKs and induction of phase 2 detoxifying enzyme activity by chlorogenic acid. *J. Biol. Chem.* 2005, 280, 27888-95.

[4]   Xu, Y.; Chen, J.; Yu, X.; Tao, W.; Jiang, F.; Yin, Z.; Liu, C. Protective effects of chlorogenic acid on acute hepatotoxicity induced by lipopolysaccharide in mice. *Inflamm. Res.* 2010, 59, 871-7.

[5]   Chauhan, P.S.; Satti, N.K.; Sharma, P.; Sharma, V.K.; Suri, K.A.; Bani, S. Differential effects of chlorogenic acid on various immunological parameters relevant to rheumatoid arthritis. *Phytother. Res.* 2012, 26, 1156-65.

[6]   Panagiotakos, D.B.; Pitsavos, C.; Chrysohoou, C.; Kokkinos, P.; Toutouzas, P.; Stefanadis, C. The J-shaped effect of coffee consumption on the risk of developing acute coronary syndromes: the CARDIO2000 case–control study. *J. Nutr.* 2003, 133, 3228–32.

[7]   Happonen, P.; Voutilainen, S.; Salonen. J.T. Coffee drinking is dose-dependently related to the risk of acute coronary events in middle-aged men. *J. Nutr.* 2004, 134, 2381–6.

[8]   Andersen, L.F.; Jacobs, Jr. D.R.; Carlsen, M.H.; Blomhoff, R. Consumption of coffee is associated with reduced risk of death attributed to inflammatory and cardiovascular diseases in the Iowa Women's Health Study. *Am. J. Clin. Nutr.* 2006, 83, 1039–46.

[9]   Watanabe, T.; Arai, Y.; Mitsui, Y.; Kusaura, T.; Okawa, W.; Kajihara, Y.; et al. The blood pressure-lowering effect and safety of chlorogenic acid from green coffee bean extract in essential hypertension. *Clin. Exp. Hypertens.* 2006, 28, 439–49.

[10]   Ochiai, R.; Jokura, H.; Suzuki, A.; Tokimutsu, I.; Ohishi, M; Komai, N., et al. Green coffee bean extract improves human vasoreactivity. *Hypertens. Res.* 2004, 27, 731–7.

[11]   Suzuki, A.; Yamamoto, N.; Jokura, H.; Yamamoto, M.; Fujii, A.; Tokimitsu, I.; et al. Chlorogenic acid attenuates hypertension and improves endothelial function in spontaneously hypertensive rats. *J. Hypertens.* 2006, 24, 1065–73.

[12]   Wu, H.Z.; Luo, J.; Yin, Y.X.; Wei, Q. Effects of chlorogenic acid, an active compound activating calcineurin, purified from Flos Lonicerae on macrophage. *Acta. Pharmacol. Sin.* 2004, 25, 1685–9.

[13] Velagaleti, R.S.; Pencina, M.J.; Murabito, J.M.; Wang, T.J.; Parikh, N.I.; D'Agostino, R.B.; Levy, D.; Kannel, W.B.; Vasan, R.S. Long-term trends in the incidence of heart failure after myocardial infarction. *Circulation.* 2008, 118, 2057-62.

[14] Onai, Y.; Suzuki, J.; Maejima, Y.; Haraguchi, G.; Muto, S.; Itai, A.; Isobe, M. Inhibition of NF-kappaB improves left ventricular remodeling and cardiac dysfunction after myocardial infarction. *Am. J. Physiol. Heart. Circ. Physiol.* 2007, 292, H530-8.

[15] Brasier, A.R. The nuclear factor-kappab-interleukin-6 signalling pathway mediating vascular inflammation. *Cardiovasc. Res.* 2010, 86, 211-8.

[16] Frangogiannis, N.G.; Smith, C.W.; Entman, M.L. The inflammatory response in myocardial infarction. *Cardiovasc. Res.* 2002, 53, 31-47.

[17] Kempf, T.; Zarbock, A.; Vestweber, D.; Wollert, K.C. Anti-inflammatory mechanisms and therapeutic opportunities in myocardial infarct healing. *J. Mol. Med. (Berl).* 2012, 90, 361-369.

[18] Vilahur, G.; Juan-Babot, O.; Pena, E.; Onate, B.; Casani, L.; Badimon, L. Molecular and cellular mechanisms involved in cardiac remodeling after acute myocardial infarction. *J. Mol. Cell. Cardiol.* 2011, 50, 522-533.

[19] Vanhoutte, D.; Schellings, M.; Pinto, Y.; Heymans, S. Relevance of matrix metalloproteinases and their inhibitors after myocardial infarction: A temporal and spatial window. *Cardiovasc. Res.* 2006, 69, 604-613.

[20] Kanno, Y.; Watanabe, R.; Zempo, H.; Ogawa, M.; Suzuki, J.; Isobe, M. Chlorogenic acid attenuates ventricular remodeling after myocardial infarction in mice. *Int. Heart. J.* 2013, 54, 176-80.

[21] Zee-Cheng, C.S.; Tsai, C.C.; Palmer, D.C.; Codd, J.E.; Pennington, D.G.; Williams, G.A. High incidence of myocarditis by endomyocardial biopsy in patients with idiopathic congestive cardiomyopathy. *J. Am. Coll. Cardiol.* 1984, 3, 63-70.

[22] Oakley, C.M. Myocarditis, pericarditis and other pericardial diseases. *Heart.* 2000, 84, 449-54.

[23] Batra, A.S.; Lewis, A.B. Acute myocarditis. *Curr. Opin. Pediatr.* 2001, 13, 234-9.

[24] Haas, G.J. Etiology, evaluation, and management of acute myocarditis. *Cardiol. Rev.* 2001, 9, 88-95.

[25] Liu, P.P.; Mason, J.W. Advances in the understanding of myocarditis. *Circulation.* 2001, 104, 1076-82.

[26] Frustaci, A.; Chimenti, C.; Calabrese, F.; Pieroni, M.; Thiene, G.; Maseri, A. Immunosuppressive therapy for active lymphocytic myocarditis: virological and immunologic profile of responders versus nonresponders. *Circulation.* 2003, 107, 857-63.

[27] Pummerer, C.L.; Luze, K.; Grassl, G.; Bachmaier, K.; Offner, F.; Burrell, S.K.; Lenz, D.M.; Zamborelli, T.J.; Penninger, J.M.; Neu, N. Identification of cardiac myosin peptides capable of inducing autoimmune myocarditis in BALB/c mice. *J. Clin. Invest.* 1996, 97, 2057-62.

[28] Suzuki, J.; Ogawa, M.; Futamatsu, H.; Kosuge, H.; Sagesaka, Y.M.; Isobe, M. Tea catechins improve left ventricular dysfunction, suppress myocardial inflammation and fibrosis, and alter cytokine expression in rat autoimmune myocarditis. *Eur. J. Heart. Fail.* 2007, 9, 152-9.

[29] Suzuki, J.; Ogawa, M.; Watanabe, R.; Morishita, R.; Hirata, Y.; Nagai, R.; Isobe, M. Autoimmune giant cell myocarditis: clinical characteristics, experimental models and future treatments. *Expert. Opin. Ther. Targets.* 2011, 15, 1163-72.

[30] Ashigaki, N.; Suzuki, J.; Ogawa, M.; Watanabe, R.; Aoyama, N.; Kobayashi, N.; Hanatani, T.; Sekinishi, A.; Zempo, H.; Tada, Y.; Takamura, C.; Wakayama, K.; Hirata, Y.; Nagai, R.; Izumi, Y.; Isobe, M. Periodontal bacteria aggravate experimental autoimmune myocarditis in mice. *Am. J. Physiol. Heart. Circ. Physiol.* 2013, 304, H740-8.

[31] Ellis, C.R.; Di Salvo, T. Myocarditis: basic and clinical aspects. *Cardiol. Rev.* 2007, 15, 170-7.

[32] Kishimoto, C.; Nimata, M.; Okabe, T.A.; Shioji, K. Immunoglobulin treatment ameliorates myocardial injury in experimental autoimmune myocarditis associated with suppression of reactive oxygen species. *Int. J. Cardiol.* 2013, 167, 140-5.

[33] Long, E.O. ICAM-1: getting a grip on leukocyte adhesion. *J. Immunol.* 2011, 186, 5021-3.

[34] Seko, Y.; Matsuda, H.; Kato, K.; Hashimoto, Y.; Yagita, H.; Okumura, K.; Yazaki, Y. Expression of intercellular adhesion molecule-1 in murine hearts with acute myocarditis caused by coxsackievirus B3. *J. Clin. Invest.* 1993, 91, 1327-36.

[35] Nakagawa, P.; Liu, Y.; Liao, T.D.; Chen, X.; Gonzalez, G.E.; Bobbitt, K.R.; Smolarek, D.; Peterson, E.L.; Kedl, R.; Yang, X.P.; Rhaleb, N.E.; Carretero, O.A. Treatment with N-acetyl-seryl-aspartyl-lysyl-proline prevents experimental autoimmune myocarditis in rats. *Am. J. Physiol. Heart. Circ. Physiol.* 2012, 303, H1114-27.

[36] Kim, Y.S.; Ahn, Y.; Hong, M.H.; Joo, S.Y.; Kim, K.H.; Sohn, I.S.; Park, H.W.; Hong, Y.J.; Kim, J.H.; Kim, W.; Jeong, M.H.; Cho, J.G.; Park, J.C.; Kang, J.C. Curcumin attenuates inflammatory responses of TNF-alpha-stimulated human endothelial cells. *J. Cardiovasc. Pharmacol.* 2007, 50, 41-9.

[37] Phalitakul, S.; Okada, M.; Hara, Y.; Yamawaki, H. Vaspin prevents TNF-alpha-induced intracellular adhesion molecule-1 via inhibiting reactive oxygen species-dependent NF-kappaB and PKCtheta activation in cultured rat vascular smooth muscle cells. *Pharmacol. Res.* 2011, 64, 493-500.

[38] Zempo, H.; Suzuki, J.; Ogawa, M.; Watanabe, R.; Tada, Y.; Takamura, C.; Isobe, M. Chlorogenic acid suppresses a cell adhesion molecule in experimental autoimmune myocarditis in mice. *Immun. Endoc. Metab. Agents in Med. Chem.* 2013, 13, 232-236.

[39] Morishita, R.; Sugimoto, T.; Aoki, M.; Kida, I.; Tomita, N.: Moriguchi, A.; Maeda, K.; Sawa, Y.; Kaneda, Y.; Higaki, J.; Ogihara, T. In vivo transfection of cis element "decoy" against nuclear factor-kappaB binding site prevents myocardial infarction. *Nat. Med.* 1997; 3: 894-899.

[40] Yokoseki, O.; Suzuki, J.; Kitabayashi, H.; Watanabe, N.; Wada, Y.; Aoki, M., Morishita, R.; Kaneda, Y.; Ogihara, T.; Futamatsu, H.; Kobayashi, Y.; Isobe, M. cis element decoy against nuclear factor-κB attenuates development of experimental autoimmune myocarditis in rats. *Circ. Res.* 2001; 89: 899-906.

[41] Suzuki, J.; Morishita, R.; Amano, J.; Kaneda, Y.; Isobe, M. Decoy against nuclear factor-kappa B attenuates myocardial cell infiltration and arterial neointimal formation in murine cardiac allografts. *Gene Ther.* 2000; 7: 1847-1852.

INDEX

A

accounting, 72
acid, ix, 16, 79, 107, 108, 111, 112, 113, 115
actin, viii, 65, 66, 67, 68, 73, 74, 78, 79, 80
active compound, 112
adhesion, 11, 110, 114, 115
adults, 91
advancement, 15, 51, 77
adventitia, 23
adverse effects, 109
age, vii, 2, 5, 6, 7, 10, 23, 24, 33, 38, 44, 56, 63, 76
albumin, 12, 13, 33, 38, 47, 57, 60, 94
aldehydes, 18
allele, 73
amino, 60, 67, 68, 69, 70, 73, 76, 79, 80
amino acid(s), 67, 68, 69, 70, 73, 76, 79, 80
amyloidosis, 14
anemia, 5, 17, 42, 46, 59
angiotensin converting enzyme, 4
angiotensin II, 19, 45, 98
antibody, 110
antihypertensive drugs, 7
antioxidant, 13, 111
aorta, 2, 6, 7, 8, 10
apoptosis, 100
arrest, 3
arrhythmia(s), 3, 109, 110

B

arterial hypertension, 9, 19, 44, 45, 63
arterial stiffness, 53, 62
arter(ies), 2, 6, 7, 9, 10, 14, 23, 35, 40, 42, 48, 50, 51, 55, 58, 62, 109
arteriosclerosis, 6, 44
assessment, 19, 21, 22, 40, 61, 62, 71
atherogenesis, 6
atherosclerosis, vii, 2, 6, 9, 10, 11, 12, 15, 16, 20, 23, 24, 35, 36, 37, 38, 39, 40, 42, 43, 44, 47, 50, 51, 54, 56, 58, 59, 62, 63, 97
atherosclerotic plaque, 6, 35, 36, 42, 62
atria, 73
autoimmune disease, 110
autosomal dominant, 72, 74, 78

bacteria, 114
base, 21
beneficial effect, x, 98, 107, 110, 111
benefits, 5
beta 2-microglobulin, 25, 33
bilateral, 23
bioavailability, 12, 48, 50, 109
biological activity, 92, 93, 94
biologically active compounds, 50
biomarkers, 14, 34, 60
biopsy, 113

C

I

J

Q

R

T

target, 87, 94, 95, 96
Task Force, 23
technical assistance, 111
tension, 45, 70, 78, 79
TGF, 99
therapeutic effect(s), 111
therapeutic interventions, 40
therapy, 7, 9, 10, 17, 21, 45, 47, 76, 114
thinning, 78
thrombosis, 12
thrombus, 70
thyroid, 95
thyroid gland, 95
tissue, 13, 15, 16, 18, 46, 62, 67, 82, 94, 99, 100
TNF-alpha, 115
tonic, 68
total cholesterol, 45
toxicity, 59
toxin, 15, 56
Tpm, viii, 65, 66, 67, 68, 69, 70, 71, 72, 73, 74, 75, 76, 78, 79, 80
traditional risk factor, vii, 1, 9, 11, 44, 52, 55
transcription, 95, 96, 99, 110
transcription factors, 96, 99, 110
transcripts, 70
transducer, 23
transfection, 115
transformation, 24
transgene, 70, 78, 85
translation, 95, 100
transmission, 78, 80
transplant, 111
transplantation, 3
transport, viii, 2, 17, 20, 36, 46, 52, 53, 61, 66, 67
transport characteristics of peritoneum, 53
transportation, 51
treatment, vii, ix, x, 1, 2, 3, 4, 6, 7, 8, 13, 17, 19, 20, 21, 22, 24, 25, 26, 28, 29, 30, 31, 32, 35, 36, 37, 38, 39, 40, 42, 43, 44, 45,

46, 47, 48, 49, 50, 51, 52, 53, 59, 77, 89, 98, 100, 107, 111, 114
trial, 21, 59, 60, 64, 86
triggers, 96
triglycerides, 33
tropomyosin, v, vii, viii, 65, 66, 67, 73, 81, 82, 83, 84, 85, 86, 87, 88
troponin, vii, viii, 2, 26, 32, 34, 35, 65, 68, 70, 71, 80, 83, 84, 86
tumor, 4, 108
tumor necrosis factor (TNF), 4, 12, 52, 108, 115

U

ultrafiltration, 19, 59
ultrasonography, 23, 42
ultrasound, vii, 1, 6, 23, 42, 43, 50, 62
United States (USA), 40, 44, 56, 57, 72, 74, 81, 82, 88, 104
urea, 22, 30, 34, 37, 51
uremia-related factors, vii, 1
Uremia-Related Risk Factors, 11
uremic, 2, 3, 4, 5, 6, 7, 8, 14, 15, 17, 24, 43, 44, 46, 52, 53, 56, 98
urine, 22, 31, 47, 49
USA, 40, 44, 57, 81, 82, 88, 104

V

validation, 61
valve, 57
valvular heart disease, 21
variables, 24
variations, 5, 34, 35, 39, 95
vascular complication, 7, 19, 44
vascular disease(s), 2, 21
vascular system, 5, 42, 43, 53
vascular wall, 7, 8
vasculature, 67, 76, 109
vasoconstriction, 12
vasodilation, 46
VCAM, 11, 12
velocity, 10, 22, 35, 43, 58